Anesthesia and Neurotoxicity

Yuji Morimoto
Editor

Anesthesia and Neurotoxicity

Springer

Editor
Yuji Morimoto
Graduate School of Medicine
Hokkaido University Graduate
School of Medicine
Sapporo
Hokkaido
Japan

ISBN 978-4-431-55623-7 ISBN 978-4-431-55624-4 (eBook)
DOI 10.1007/978-4-431-55624-4

Library of Congress Control Number: 2017943096

Printed on acid-free paper

This Springer imprint is published by Springer Nature
The registered company is Springer Japan KK
The registered company address is: Chiyoda First Bldg. East, 3-8-1 Nishi-Kanda, Chiyoda-ku, Tokyo 101-0065, Japan

Preface

Recent progress in the field of medicine, especially in surgery, has made it possible to save many lives that previously would have been lost. Advances in anesthesiology have greatly supported this progression. The estimated annual number of procedures employing general anesthesia in Japan has already reached approximately three million, and general anesthetics are no longer considered to be special drugs.

Anesthetics used for analgesia and sedation can nullify pain and free patients from the fear of surgery. In addition, their effects are so rapid as to be almost instantaneous. Accordingly, it is no exaggeration to say that they are extremely strong drugs, more potent than any others. Therefore, it is not strange to think that they have effects other than the anesthetic one on the whole body. Above all, we anesthesiologists have continued to entertain the "sweet dream" that anesthetics are protective for many organs. In the central nervous system, there have been innumerable studies on protection of the brain and spinal cord by anesthetics, and animal studies strongly support these ideas. However, these effects have not yet been proven for humans in clinical practice.

On the other hand, after the 1990s, a negative side of anesthetics, neurotoxicity, began to attract attention. Neurotoxic effects were noted for local anesthetics, NMDA receptor blockers such as nitrous oxide or ketamine, and opioids, which were observed to affect the spinal cord. Recently, neurotoxicity for the developing brain, postoperative delirium (POD), and postoperative cognitive dysfunction (POCD) are well known.

With regard to neurotoxicity for the developing brain, this problem began to be widely discussed after the famous paper by Jevtovic-Todorovic et al. in 2003 (J Neurosci 23: 876–882, 2003). Since their report, the number of articles about the neurotoxicity of anesthetics in developing animals (mainly rodents) has increased year by year. Now it is widely accepted that most anesthetics are neurotoxic to the developing animal brain.

Actually, POD and POCD have long been known to many anesthesiologists as a result of their experiences in clinical practice. However, worldwide interest in them grew after the report of the multicenter study by the International Study of Postoperative Cognitive Dysfunction group (ISPOCD) in 1998 (Lancet 351:857–861, 1998). Thus, many studies on the basic and clinical aspects of these conditions have now been reported.

In this book, Japanese authorities in the field of neuroanesthesia, including the neurotoxicity of anesthetics, review these two hot topics. I sincerely hope that this book will benefit both clinicians and researchers, not only those who are anesthesiologists, but also pediatricians, obstetricians, surgeons, basic researchers, and others.

Sapporo, Hokkaido, Japan Yuji Morimoto M.D., Ph.D.

Contents

Part I Neurotoxicity of the Anesthetics for Developing Brain

1 **Laboratory Findings: To What Degree Can We Extrapolate the Animal Data to the Bedside?** 3
Yuji Morimoto, Yosuke Uchida, and Hitoshi Saito

2 **Clinical Findings Including Prevention and Treatment** 17
Yasushi Satoh

3 **Implications for Pediatric Anesthesia** 33
Koichi Yuki, Yasushi Mio, and Shoichi Uezono

Part II Postoperative Delirium and Cognitive Dysfunction

4 **Present Clinical Status of Postoperative Delirium (POD)** 51
Moritoki Egi

5 **Present Clinical Status of Postoperative Cognitive Dysfunction in Cardiovascular Surgery** 59
Kazuyoshi Ishida, Atsuo Yamashita, Satoshi Yamashita, and Mishiya Matsumoto

6 **Present Clinical Status of Postoperative Cognitive Dysfunction Following Noncardiac Surgery** 95
Tatsuo Horiuchi, Tomonori Takazawa, and Shigeru Saito

7 **Diagnosis of POD and POCD** 105
Shigehito Sawamura

8 **Prevention and Treatment of Postoperative Delirium and Postoperative Cognitive Dysfunction** 121
Mitsuru Ida and Masahiko Kawaguchi

9 Mechanisms of POD and POCD: Effects of Anesthetics 133
Tomoyuki Miyazaki, Yoshikazu Yamaguchi, and Takahisa Goto

10 Mechanism of POD and POCD - Effect of Other Than Anesthetics 151
Shusuke Sekine and Hiroyuki Uchino

Part I
Neurotoxicity of the Anesthetics for Developing Brain

Chapter 1
Laboratory Findings: To What Degree Can We Extrapolate the Animal Data to the Bedside?

Yuji Morimoto, Yosuke Uchida, and Hitoshi Saito

Abstract After the "famous" paper by Jevtovic-Todorovic et al. published in the *Journal of Neuroscience* in 2003, the number of articles about the neurotoxicity of anesthetics in developing animals has increased year by year. Thus, it is no exaggeration to say that most anesthetics are neurotoxic to the developing animal brain. The mechanism was first suggested to be neuronal apoptosis, and then abnormality of neurotransmission, especially the manipulation of the GABAergic system during the most intense phase of synaptogenesis. Recently, based on various animal studies, many hypotheses have been reported. However, this finding has not been proven in humans yet. Moreover, the clinical impression that anesthesia has a negative effect on the neurological development of infants and children seems extremely rare for the clinician. Thus, there seem to be big discrepancies between the findings for animals and humans. The reasons for this are hypothesized to be respiratory depression caused by anesthetics, the absence of noxious stimulation during neonatal animal experiments, and the differences of the life span (that is, the length of anesthetic time) and the period of the brain growth spurt between humans and animals. Accordingly, we are now awaiting the results of several ongoing prospective clinical studies to determine whether anesthetics are really neurotoxic to the developing human brain.

Keywords Nerotoxicity • Developing • Anesthetics • Apoptosis • Synaptogenesis • Brain growth spurt

---

Y. Morimoto (✉) • Y. Uchida • H. Saito
Department of Anesthesiology & Critical Care Medicine, Hokkaido University Graduate School of Medicine, N15 W7, Kita-ku, Sapporo, Hokkaido 060-0815, Japan
e-mail: morim2@med.hokudai.ac.jp

Y. Morimoto (ed.), *Anesthesia and Neurotoxicity*,
DOI 10.1007/978-4-431-55624-4_1

Table 1.1 Anesthetics that were reported to have neurotoxicity for the developing animal brain

Inhalation anesthetics
Halothane, isoflurane, sevoflurane, desflurane
Nitrous oxide
Xenon
Intravenous anesthetics
Ketamine
Propofol
Barbiturates
Benzodiazepines
Morphine (maternal administration)

1.1 History and the Present Situation

In the 1980s, it was already reported that exposure to halothane caused neurotoxicity to the developing rat brain. However, this attracted little attention, partly because the exposure period was very long, such as during gestation and for 60 days after birth [1]. This problem came to attract great attention after the "famous" paper by Jevtovic-Todorovic et al. in 2003 [2]. Before then, their laboratory group examined the effects of ethanol on the developing human brain as a mechanism of fetal alcohol syndrome [3]. They clarified that ethanol triggered widespread apoptotic neurodegeneration in the developing rat forebrain. Because ethanol has dual actions (blockade of *N*-methyl-D-aspartate [NMDA] glutamate receptors and excessive activation of $GABA_A$ receptors), they speculated that anesthetic agents having the same actions might cause neurotoxicity in the developing brain. Then they administered a combination of anesthetics commonly used in pediatric anesthesia (midazolam, nitrous oxide, and isoflurane) to 7-day-old infant rats for 6 h and observed that this caused widespread apoptotic neurodegeneration in the developing brain, deficits in hippocampal synaptic function, and persistent memory/learning impairments [2]. It is known that midazolam and isoflurane are activators of $GABA_A$ receptors and that nitrous oxide blockades NMDA receptors. After their report, the number of articles about the neurotoxicity of anesthetics to developing animals (mainly rodents) has increased year by year. Now it is no exaggeration to say that most anesthetics are neurotoxic to the developing animal brain (Table 1.1).

1.2 Mechanism

1.2.1 Apoptosis

As mentioned above, the mechanism assumed first was apoptotic neurodegeneration through the blockade of NMDA receptors and activation of $GABA_A$ receptors. Olney et al. proposed that the blockade of NMDA receptors and activation of $GABA_A$ receptors abnormally inhibited neurons and induced translocation of BAX protein to mitochondrial membranes, where it would disrupt membrane permeability, allowing extramitochondrial leakage of cytochrome C (the so-called apoptotic cascade) [4]. The mechanisms that mediate Bax translocation to mitochondrial membranes remain elusive, but mitogen-activated plasma kinase systems, especially the extracellular signal regulated protein kinase (ERK) pathway, have been implicated [5]. However, it has been reported that ketamine (a blocker of NMDA receptors) alone [6] and propofol (an activator of $GABA_A$ receptors) alone [7] cause apoptosis in the developing rodent brain, demonstrating that dual action is not absolutely necessary to induce apoptosis. Moreover, Stratmann et al. evaluated isoflurane-induced neurotoxicity along with the effect of hypercapnia [8]. The degree and distribution of thalamic cell death were similar in isoflurane-treated and carbon dioxide-treated rats. However, only 4 h of isoflurane caused a long-term neurocognitive deficit. This indicates that there is inconsistency between cell death during the developing stage and the neurocognitive outcome in the adult. Actually, as many as 50–70% of neurons and progenitor cells undergo physiological cell death and elimination by apoptosis during normal CNS development because neurons are produced in excess at this stage [5, 9]. Accordingly, apoptotic neuronal cell death induced by anesthetics may be involved in the physiological cell death during the developing stage.

1.2.2 Abnormalities of Neural Transmission

In addition to neurons, many more synapses are formed throughout the developing stage. Then reorganization of synapse formation, including synaptic pruning and switching of neurotransmission, occurs to achieve plasticity and stabilization of the circuits [10, 11]. The most intense phase of synaptogenesis is referred to as the brain growth spurt and is species dependent [10]. In the rodent cerebral cortex, this period is limited to a narrow time window between the second and fourth postnatal weeks, which coincide with the period of vulnerability to anesthetics. Because anesthetics act on receptors and/or ion channels, they may be able to modulate synaptic formation during the brain growth spurt.

The following section discusses our study examining the effects of neonatal pentobarbital exposure on long-term hippocampal synaptic plasticity [12]. On postnatal day 7 (P 7), pentobarbital (10 or 20 mg/kg) was administered intraperitoneally to rats. Exposure to pentobarbital caused significant suppression of long-term potentiation (LTP) induction in the postgrowth period (Fig. 1.1). In the same experimental system, we evaluated the effects of sevoflurane [13] and propofol (data not published), both of which are known as GABAergic anesthetics, as well as pentobarbital and clarified that neonatal exposure to these drugs inhibited LTP induction after growth. In addition, paired-pulse stimulation in the population spikes later in adulthood was tested in the pentobarbital-treated rats [12] (Fig. 1.2). These rats showed reduced paired-pulse inhibition, which indicated that neonatal manipulation of GABA receptors by pentobarbital caused persistent reduction of GABAergic inhibition in hippocampal synapses in adults. The reduction of GABAergic inhibi-

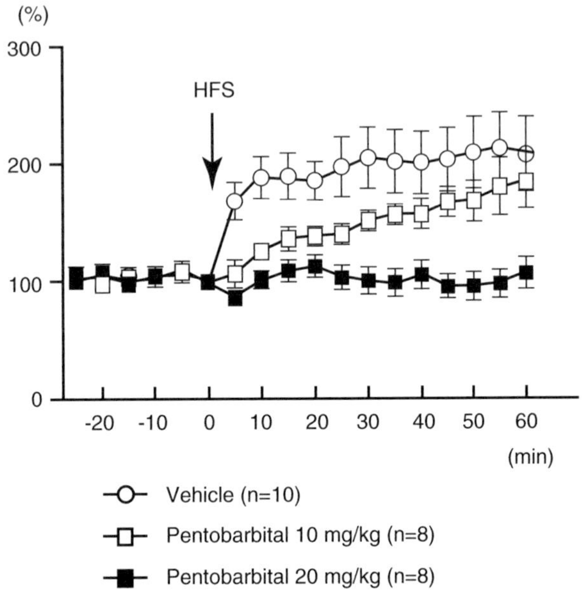

Fig. 1.1 Time course response of population spike amplitude (PSA) during the 60 min after high-frequency stimulation (HFS) in the postgrowth period after neonatal exposure to pentobarbital (modified from Brain Res 2011; 1388:69–76). At 10 mg/kg, pentobarbital suppressed the initial induction of LTP; however, PSA was gradually augmented within 60 min of observation. At 20 mg/kg, LTP induction was completely suppressed

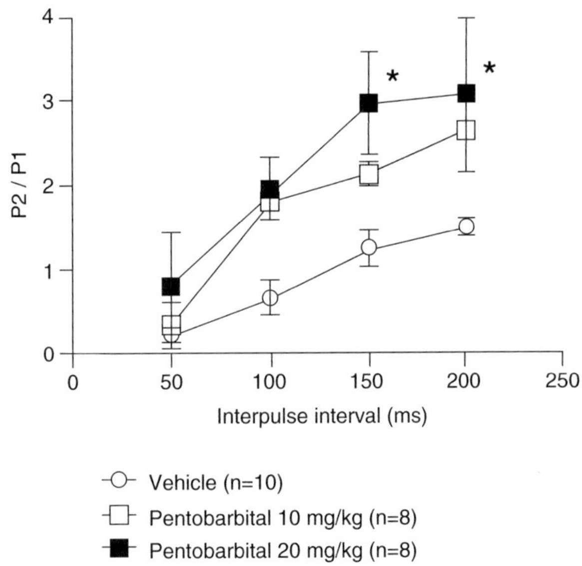

Fig. 1.2 Hippocampal paired-pulse response in the population spikes later in adulthood (modified from Brain Res 2011; 1388:69–76). Both pentobarbital treatment groups showed no inhibition, but rather clear facilitation of the second population spike at stimulation strength. $^{*}P < 0.05$ vs. vehicle group

tion by neonatal GABA manipulation can increase the excitability of the pyramidal cells, which might induce the suppression of LTP due to its occlusion or saturation [12]. Another recent study evaluated the synapse density by electron microscopy after neonatal exposure to propofol [14]. Exposure of rat pups to propofol at P 5 and 10 significantly decreased dendritic spine density, whereas this drug induced a significant increase in the spine density when administered at P 15, 20, or 30. These modifications in dendritic spine densities persisted up to postnatal day 90. Another study evaluated the effects of anesthetics on axon guidance using rodent cortex brain slices and isolated neuron assays [15]. Axon guidance is an important process by which neurons send out axons to reach the correct targets. Isoflurane exposure caused errors in Semaphorin-3A-dependent axon targeting at clinically relevant anesthetic doses of numerous anesthetics acting on $GABA_A$ receptors such as sevoflurane, desflurane, thiopental, and propofol, and was reproduced with a selective agonist for it. On the other hand, nitrous oxide, fentanyl, dexmedetomidine, and ketamine had no effects. Indeed, GABAergic neurotransmission is initially excitatory and then moves to inhibition during the second postnatal week in the rodent cerebral cortex [10, 16]. In the immature neuron, the intracellular Cl^- concentration is high due to the expression of the N^+-K^+-$2Cl^-$ cotransporter NKCC1, the ability of which to extrude Cl^- toward the outside is weak. Therefore, an efflux of Cl^- occurs via opening of the Cl^- channel through the GABA agonist. In contrast, the developmental switch to the expression of the K^+-Cl^- cotransporter KCC2 lowers the intracellular Cl^- concentration due to its high ability to extrude Cl^- toward the outside. After that, the reverse phenomenon is induced by GABA agonists. Thus, the excitatory effect by GABAergic anesthetics might disturb normal synaptic formation in the immature brain. In the study mentioned above, exposure of rat pups to propofol before P 10 significantly decreased dendritic spine density, whereas a significant increase in spine density occurred after P 15, 20, and 30 [14]. This suggests that the effect of propofol changes from excitatory to inhibitory at around P 10–15.

What, then, about the participation of NMDA receptors in neural transmission? There have been many reports that ketamine causes apoptosis in the developing brain [6, 17]. However, as far as we know, few studies have evaluated the effect of ketamine on synaptogenesis. In one study using rat hippocampal slices, S(+)-ketamine exerted a toxic effect through the suppression of neuronal Ca^{2+} oscillations, which are present during a time period with high neuronal plasticity, downregulation of CaMKII, and consecutively reduced synaptic integrity [18]. In another study, the effect of ketamine–xylazine ($\alpha 2$ adrenergic agonists) anesthesia on motor learning-induced synaptic remodeling was examined in vivo by repeatedly imaging fluorescently labeled postsynaptic dendritic spines in the mouse primary motor cortex [19]. Three exposures to this anesthetic between P 14 and P 18 impaired the animals' motor learning and learning-dependent dendritic spine plasticity without cell apoptosis. The authors speculated that ketamine-induced NMDA receptor inactivation could significantly reduce activity-mediated Ca^{2+} influx into neurons, which in turn would affect synapse formation and plasticity.

To investigate the participation of $\alpha 2$ adrenergic receptors, we studied the long-term effects of neonatal administration of dexmedetomidine (DEX) on hippocampal synaptic activity by evaluating LTP induction and paired-pulse stimulation in the postgrowth period [20]. DEX-treated rats showed no impairment in the induction of LTP. Furthermore, the response in population spikes to the paired stimuli was not impaired by neonatal administration of DEX.

1.2.3 *Other Mechanisms*

1.2.3.1 Mitochondrial Injury

Mitochondria are cell organelles that are constantly remodeling via fusion and fission. For rats, it was reported that exposure to general anesthesia (midazolam, nitrous oxide, and isoflurane) at P 7 caused injury to the mitochondria at P 21, including enlargement [21]. This indicated the predominance of fusion, impairment of structural integrity, an increase in their complex IV activity, and decrease in their regional distribution in presynaptic neuronal profiles, where their presence is important for the normal development and functioning of synapses. Indeed, this study showed that inhibitory neurotransmission was impaired in the subiculum at P 21-8. Subsequently, the same group demonstrated that early exposure to the same combination of general anesthesia at P 7 caused acute reactive oxygen species upregulation and disturbed the fine balance between mitochondrial fission and fusion, leading to excessive fission and disturbed mitochondrial morphogenesis at P 8 [22]. They concluded that these effects might be related to neuronal apoptosis.

1.2.3.2 Contribution of Brain-Derived Neurotrophic Factor (BDNF) (Fig. 1.3)

BDNF supports the survival of existing neurons and encourages the growth and differentiation of new neurons and synapses. proBDNF is cleaved into mature BDNF (mBDNF) by plasmin, a protease converted from plasminogen by tissue plasminogen activator (tPA) that is released with neuronal activity. It has been reported that isoflurane reduces synaptic tPA release and increases proBDNF, which induces neuronal apoptosis and synaptic loss through the enhancement of p75 neurotrophic receptor ($p75^{NTR}$) signaling in the rodent developing brain [23]. Additional work has indicated that the $p75^{NTR}$ receptor activates RhoA, a small guanosine triphosphate that induces cytoskeletal depolymerization and apoptosis [24]. The same group has reported that propofol has the same action in the developing neuron [25].

1.2.3.3 Granule Cell Ectopia

Recently, it was reported that excitatory $GABA_A$ receptor signaling was enhanced after febrile seizures and disturbed the radical migration of neonatally generated granules cells, resulting in persistent granule cell ectopia [26]. Accordingly, we hypothesized that neonatal exposure to GABAergic anesthetics might cause granule

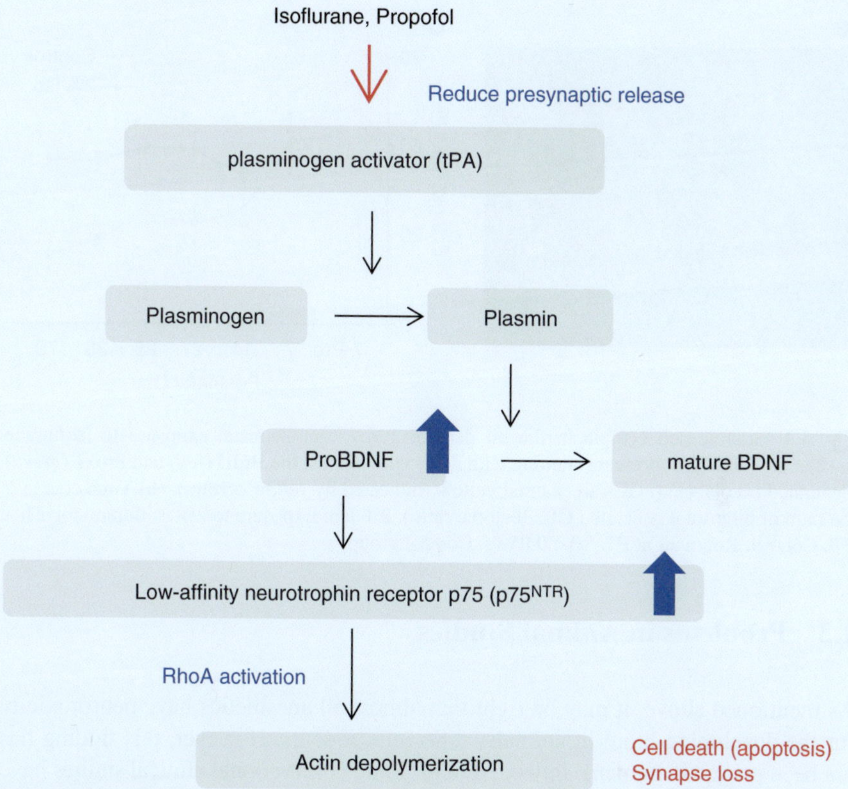

Fig. 1.3 Contribution of brain-derived neurotrophic factor (BDNF) to the neurotoxicity in the developing brain (modified from Anesthesiology 2009; 110:813–25, Anesthesiology 2011; 114:49–57, and Anesthesiology 2012; 116:352–61)

cell ectopia in the rat dentate gyrus. The example of isoflurane follows. Rat pups were subcutaneously injected with 5-bromo-2′-deoxyuridine (BrdU), a marker of cell proliferation, to label the newborn granule cells (GCs) at P 6. Then the rats were exposed to 2% isoflurane. At several time points after the exposure, double immunofluorescent staining with antibodies against BrdU and homeobox prospero-like protein 1 (Prox1) as a marker of GCs was performed to examine the localization of BrdU/Prox1 colabeled cells by confocal microscopy. The ratio of hilar/total colabeled GCs (ectopic ratio) was calculated and found to significantly increase after P21 (Fig. 1.4). Thus, it is possible that neonatal exposure to GABAergic anesthetics causes aberrant migration of the granule cells and then morphologic abnormalities after growth.

In addition to the above, many hypotheses, including neuroinflammation [27] and downregulation of microRNA [28], have been reported.

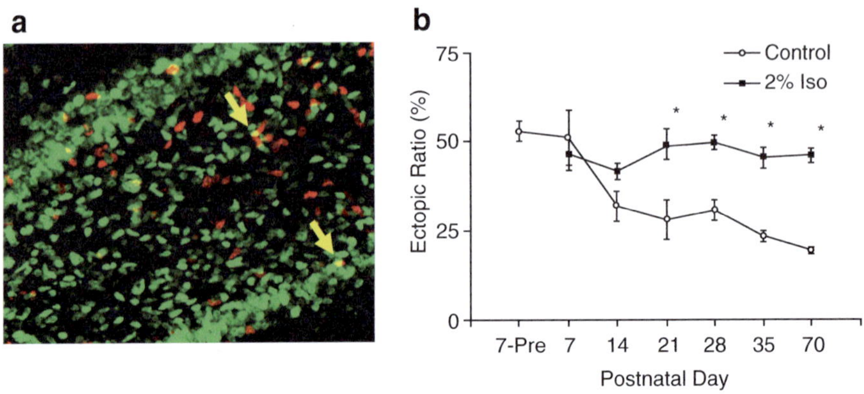

Fig. 1.4 Granule cell ectopia in the rat dentate gyrus after neonatal exposure to isoflurane. (**a**) Double immunofluorescent staining with antibodies against the BrdU (*red*) and Prox1 (*green*). Generated (=colabeled) GCs are stained yellow (indicated by *yellow arrows*). (**b**) Time course of the ratio of hilar/total generated GCs (ectopic ratio). 2% Iso: Exposure to 2% isoflurane for 2 h at P 7. Control: Room air at P7. **P* < 0.05 vs. Control group

1.3 Problems in Animal Studies

As mentioned above, it may be right that almost all anesthetics have neurotoxicity for the developing brain in animals, especially rodents. However, this finding has not been proven in humans. Indeed, though some observational clinical studies have supported this finding [29, 30], it is very difficult to separate the effects of anesthesia from surgery and comorbidity in these studies. Moreover, the clinical impression that anesthesia has a negative effect on neurological development in infants and children seems to be extremely rare among clinicians, including anesthesiologists. Thus, there seem to be big discrepancies between findings for animals and humans. We will discuss the causes of these below.

1.3.1 Respiratory Depression by Anesthetics

Airway management such as tracheal intubation and mechanical ventilation is very difficult during experiments using neonatal animals. However, many previous reports stated that blood gas data were within normal ranges. On the other hand, some reports demonstrated respiratory depression by anesthetics such as hypercapnia and hypoxia, including our laboratory data [8, 12, 13]. For example, intraperitoneal administration of 20 mg of pentobarbital to P 7 neonatal rats under room air causes severe hypercapnia at a $PaCO_2$ of around 90 mmHg and moderate hypoxia at a PaO_2 of around 50 mmHg, accompanied by metabolic acidosis [12]. Administration of 2% sevoflurane to P 7 neonatal rats under 98% oxygen also causes severe

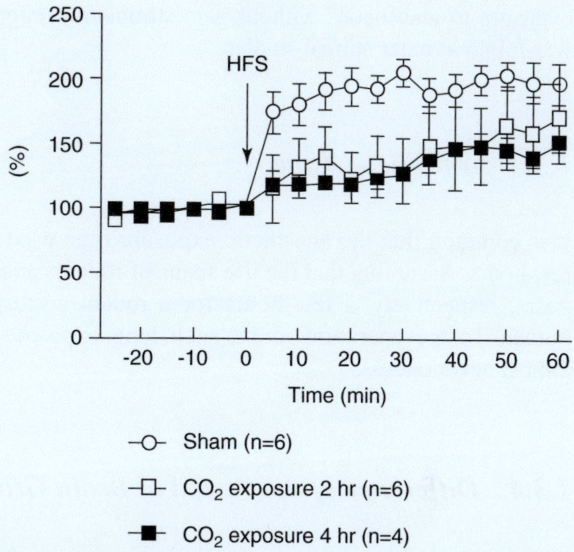

Fig. 1.5 Time course response of PSA during the 60 min after HFS in the postgrowth period after neonatal exposure to a high concentration of carbon dioxide (modified from Brain Res 2013; 1507:83–90)

hypercapnia at a $PaCO_2$ of around 80 mmHg without hypoxia [13]. Accordingly, we examined the effect of hypercapnia with hypoxia and metabolic acidosis to simulate the effect of administration of 20 mg of pentobarbital [31]. For this, neonatal P 7 rats were exposed to 13% carbon dioxide. As a result, LTP induction in the synapses of the hippocampal CA1 area was impaired later in adulthood (Fig. 1.5). Learning acquisition assessed by the Morris water maze test was also disrupted in adulthood. In another study, P14 rats were assigned to spontaneous breathing (SB) or mechanical ventilation (MV) under sevoflurane or isoflurane [32]. The rats with SB developed hypercapnia, hypoxia, and low blood pressure. Mortality and neuronal death in the hippocampus in the SB group were significantly higher than in the MV group. The rats in the SB group performed worse on the Morris water maze test 2 weeks after the anesthesia. Thus, there is a possibility that respiratory depression induced by anesthetics affects the results seen in neurotoxicity experiments in the newborn rodent model.

1.3.2 Effect of Concurrent Noxious Stimulation

Animal neurotoxicity studies are commonly performed in isolation without concurrent noxious stimulation, a condition that does not reflect the interaction of anesthesia and surgical stimulation. Therefore, an experiment in which P 7 rats were randomized into groups with exposure to ketamine with and without peripheral noxious stimulation by intraplantar injection of complete Freund's adjuvant was performed [33]. It was found that ketamine increased neuroapoptosis and simultaneous peripheral noxious stimulation reduced it. This study suggested that single exposure to anesthetics without pain stimulation might enhance neurotoxicity as was found in other animal studies.

1.3.3 Anesthetic Time

It is common that the anesthetic exposure time used in animal experiments is a few hours. Assuming that the life spans of rodents and human beings are 3 and 75 years, respectively, a few hours for a rodent corresponds to a few days for a human. In the operation room, such long exposure of children to anesthetics almost never occurs.

1.3.4 Difference of the Period of Brain Growth Spurt

As mentioned above, the period of the brain growth spurt in rodents is thought to be between the second and fourth postnatal weeks [10]. On the other hand, in humans it is thought to occur during the last trimester and up to 3 years postnatally [30]. However, a more contemporary neuroinformatics approach combining neuroscience, evolutionary science, statistical modeling, and computer science to compare brain development among different species suggested that the brain developmental state of a newborn, P 7 rat more closely corresponds to the human fetus between 17 and 22 weeks of gestation [34]. Moreover, it was reported that when pregnant rodents at gestation day 14 (corresponding to the second trimester in humans) were exposed to isoflurane [35] or sevoflurane [36] their offspring showed neurological deficits after growth. These studies suggest that neurotoxicity may also occur before the brain growth spurt in rodents. We have been very concerned with the effect of anesthesia on small children, especially those under 3 years of age [37]. However, this problem may, in fact, be mainly related to fetuses. Recently, fetal surgery is conducted for congenital diaphragmatic hernias, congenital pulmonary adenomatoid malformation, congenital heart disease, and so on [38]. Fetal cardiac depression and bradycardia have been frequently observed during fetal surgery, especially with high concentrations of inhalational anesthetics, which may increase the risk of neurological injuries [39]. However, the effects of anesthetics per se remain unknown. Moreover, when we consider the difference of anesthetic times in addition to the difference of the period of the brain growth spurt, the situation closest to the clinical setting may be the long sedation of premature babies. However, as far as we know, there have been few studies to evaluate the effects of prolonged use of sedative agents on premature babies. In one French multicenter study, the presence of moderate or severe disability at 5 years of age was prospectively evaluated after prolonged (more than 7 days) exposure to sedative and/or analgesic drugs in very preterm infants with gestational ages of fewer than 33 weeks [40]. The results indicated that such treatments were not associated with a poor 5-year neurological outcome after adjustment for the propensity score compared to infants without treatment.

1.4 Conclusions

What we want to emphasize most is that this topic arose from animal findings, not from clinical problems. It is hard to find clinical reports that clearly demonstrate a human baby suffered from a poorer neurological outcome such as learning disability due to the effect of anesthetics themselves. As mentioned above, it is supposed that almost all the anesthesiologists in the world have no clinical impression that anesthesia directly causes a negative effect on the neurological development of infants and children. Recently, it was reported that even the most promising findings from animal research often fail in human trials and are rarely adopted into clinical practice [41]. For example, in stroke medicine, animal models have failed to yield a single neuroprotective treatment for humans, although there have been numerous positive animal data. Our first clear knowledge of whether anesthetics are really neurotoxic to the human developing brain will come from the results of several ongoing prospective clinical studies [30].

References

1. Uemura E, Levin ED, Bowman RE (1985) Effects of halothane on synaptogenesis and learning behavior in rats. Exp Neurol 89:520–529
2. Jevtovic-Todorovic V, Hartman RE, Izumi Y et al (2003) Early exposure to common anesthetic agents causes widespread neurodegeneration in the developing rat brain and persistent learning deficits. J Neurosci 23:876–882
3. Ikonomidou C, Bittigau P, Ishimaru MJ et al (2000) Ethanol-induced apoptotic neurodegeneration and fetal alcohol syndrome. Science 287:1056–1060
4. Olney JW, Young C, Wozniak DF et al (2004) Anesthesia-induced developmental neuroapoptosis. Does it happen in humans? Anesthesiology 101:273–275
5. Creeley CE, Olney JW (2010) The young: neuroapoptosis induced by anesthetics and what to do about it. Anesth Analg 110:442–448
6. Soriano SG, Liu Q, Li J et al (2010) Ketamine activates cell cycle signaling and apoptosis in the neonatal rat brain. Anesthesiology 112:1155–1163
7. Cattano D, Young C, Straiko MM et al (2008) Subanesthetic doses of propofol induce neuroapoptosis in the infant mouse brain. Anesth Analg 106:1712–1714
8. Stratmann G, May LD, Sall JW et al (2009) Effect of hypercarbia and isoflurane on brain cell death and neurocognitive dysfunction in 7-day-old rats. Anesthesiology 110:849–861
9. Loepke AW, Soriano SG (2008) An assessment of the effects of general anesthetics on developing brain structure and neurocognitive function. Anesth Analg 106:1681–1707
10. Vutskits L (2012) General anesthesia: a gateway to modulate synapse formation and neural plasticity? Anesth Analg 115:1174–1182
11. Perouansky M, Hemmings HC Jr (2009) Neurotoxicity of general anesthetics: cause for concern? Anesthesiology 111:1365–1371

12. Tachibana K, Hashimoto T, Kato R et al (2011) Long-lasting effects of neonatal pentobarbital administration on spatial learning and hippocampal synaptic plasticity. Brain Res 1388:69–76
13. Kato R, Tachibana K, Nishimoto N et al (2013) Neonatal exposure to sevoflurane causes significant suppression of hippocampal long-term potentiation in postgrowth rats. Anesth Analg 117:1429–1435
14. Briner A, Nikonenko I, De Roo M et al (2011) Developmental stage-dependent persistent impact of propofol anesthesia on dendritic spines in the rat medial prefrontal cortex. Anesthesiology 115:282–293
15. Mintz CD, Barrett KM, Smith SC et al (2013) Anesthetics interfere with axon guidance in developing mouse neocortical neurons in vitro via a -aminobutyric acid type A receptor mechanism. Anesthesiology 118:825–833
16. Ben-Ari Y (2002) Excitatory actions of gaba during development: the nature of the nurture. Nat Rev Neurosci 3:728–739
17. Brambrink AM, Evers AS, Avidan MS et al (2012) Ketamine-induced neuroapoptosis in the fetal and neonatal rhesus macaque brain. Anesthesiology 116:372–384
18. Sinner B, Friedrich O, Zink W et al (2011) The toxic effects of s(+)-ketamine on differentiating neurons in vitro as a consequence of suppressed neuronal Ca2+ oscillations. Anesth Analg 113:1161–1169
19. Huang L, Yang G (2015) Repeated exposure to ketamine-xylazine during early development impairs motor learning-dependent dendritic spine plasticity in adulthood. Anesthesiology 122:821–831
20. Tachibana K, Hashimoto T, Kato R et al (2012) Neonatal administration with dexmedetomidine does not impair the rat hippocampal synaptic plasticity later in adulthood. Paediatr Anaesth 22:713–719
21. Sanchez V, Feinstein SD, Lunardi N et al (2011) General anesthesia causes long-term impairment of mitochondrial morphogenesis and synaptic transmission in developing rat brain. Anesthesiology 115:992–1002
22. Boscolo A, Milanovic D, Starr JA et al (2013) Early exposure to general anesthesia disturbs mitochondrial fission and fusion in the developing rat brain. Anesthesiology 118:1086–1097
23. Head BP, Patel HH, Niesman IR et al (2009) Inhibition of p75 neurotrophin receptor attenuates isoflurane-mediated neuronal apoptosis in the neonatal central nervous system. Anesthesiology 110:813–825
24. Lemkuil BP, Head BP, Pearn ML et al (2011) Isoflurane neurotoxicity is mediated by p75NTR-RhoA activation and actin depolymerization. Anesthesiology 114:49–57
25. Pearn ML, Hu Y, Niesman IR et al (2012) Propofol neurotoxicity is mediated by p75 neurotrophin receptor activation. Anesthesiology 116:352–361
26. Koyama R, Tao K, Sasaki T et al (2012) GABAergic excitation after febrile seizures induces ectopic granule cells and adult epilepsy. Nat Med 18:1271–1278
27. Shen X, Dong Y, Xu Z et al (2013) Selective anesthesia-induced neuroinflammation in developing mouse brain and cognitive impairment. Anesthesiology 118:502–515
28. Twaroski DM, Yan Y, Olson JM et al (2014) Down-regulation of microRNA-21 is involved in the propofol-induced neurotoxicity observed in human stem cell-derived neurons. Anesthesiology 121:786–800
29. Sinner B, Becke K, Engelhard K (2014) General anaesthetics and the developing brain: an overview. Anaesthesia 69:1009–1022
30. Hansen TG (2015) Anesthesia-related neurotoxicity and the developing animal brain is not a significant problem in children. Paediatr Anaesth 25:65–72
31. Tachibana K, Hashimoto T, Takita K et al (2013) Neonatal exposure to high concentration of carbon dioxide produces persistent learning deficits with impaired hippocampal synaptic plasticity. Brain Res 1507:83–90
32. Wu B, Yu Z, You S et al (2014) Physiological disturbance may contribute to neurodegeneration induced by isoflurane or sevoflurane in 14 day old rats. PLoS One 9:e84622

33. Liu JR, Liu Q, Li J et al (2012) Noxious stimulation attenuates ketamine-induced neuroapoptosis in the developing rat brain. Anesthesiology 117:64–71
34. Loepke AW, McGowan FX Jr, Soriano SG (2008) CON: the toxic effects of anesthetics in the developing brain: the clinical perspective. Anesth Analg 106:1664–1669
35. Palanisamy A, Baxter MG, Keel PK et al (2011) Rats exposed to isoflurane in utero during early gestation are behaviorally abnormal as adults. Anesthesiology 114:521–528
36. Zheng H, Dong Y, Xu Z et al (2013) Sevoflurane anesthesia in pregnant mice induces neurotoxicity in fetal and offspring mice. Anesthesiology 118:516–526
37. Rappaport BA, Suresh S, Hertz S et al (2015) Anesthetic neurotoxicity—clinical implications of animal models. N Engl J Med 372:796–797
38. Sala P, Prefumo F, Pastorino D et al (2014) Fetal surgery: an overview. Obstet Gynecol Surv 69:218–228
39. Boat AC, Sadhasivam S, Loepke AW et al (2011) Outcome for the extremely premature neonate: how far do we push the edge? Paediatr Anaesth 21:765–770
40. Roze JC, Denizot S, Carbajal R et al (2008) Prolonged sedation and/or analgesia and 5-year neurodevelopment outcome in very preterm infants: results from the EPIPAGE cohort. Arch Pediatr Adolesc Med 162:728–733
41. Pound P, Bracken MB (2014) Is animal research sufficiently evidence based to be a cornerstone of biomedical research? BMJ 348:g3387

Chapter 2
Clinical Findings Including Prevention and Treatment

Yasushi Satoh

Abstract Scientific and public attention to the potential neurodevelopmental effects of anesthesia during early childhood has been increasing considerably. In February 2015, the New York Times published an article to inform parents of potential issues with anesthesia use among young children. Parents whose children need surgery are increasingly questioning anesthesiologists regarding this issue. However, associations between anesthesia exposure during infancy and adverse neurodevelopmental outcomes have not been definitively demonstrated in existing studies. In this chapter, the clinical findings on this issue are summarized and the prevention and treatment that contribute to the management of this issue are reviewed.

Keywords Neurotoxicity • Neurodevelopment • Children • General anesthetics

2.1 Introduction

In 1945, Levy reported postoperative behavioral changes in children under the age of 3 [1]. These children exhibited sleep and eating disorders, separation anxiety, temper tantrums, and aggression toward authorities, which were estimated to occur in up to 60% of all children exposed to general anesthesia. However, these observations pertained to short-term changes after exposure to anesthesia.

The concern about long-term neurodevelopmental changes has arisen from a laboratory study published in 2003. Jevtovic-Todorovic et al. reported that general anesthesia administered to a 7-day-old rat caused apoptosis in the brain and a learning

Y. Satoh
Department of Pharmacology, National Defense Medical College,
Tokorozawa, Saitama 359-8513, Japan

Department of Anesthesiology, National Defense Medical College,
Tokorozawa, Saitama 359-8513, Japan
e-mail: wndlt3@gmail.com

Y. Morimoto (ed.), *Anesthesia and Neurotoxicity*,
DOI 10.1007/978-4-431-55624-4_2

disability in adulthood [2]. After this study, a growing body of evidence indicates that almost all general anesthetics cause long-term behavioral abnormalities in young animals, including rodents and subhuman primates (see Chap. 1). These changes include not only learning disabilities but also social deficits related to the autism spectrum disorder (ASD) [3]. It remains unclear if similar outcomes would occur in humans but concern is growing regarding the safety of pediatric and obstetric anesthetics. This was the rare instance that the results of a laboratory study prompted a clinical study. It is estimated that 1.5 million infants receive anesthesia for surgical procedures each year in the USA alone [4]. Therefore, this issue is an important and urgent matter of public health. Should general anesthesia have deleterious effects for the developing brain, we must develop alternative strategies to anesthetize young children, including novel anesthetic agents with an alternative mechanism of action and minimal neurotoxicity.

The concerns of the US Food and Drug Administration (FDA) on this issue initiated a nonprofit public-private partnership project with the International Anesthesia Research Society (IARS) called "Strategies for Mitigating Anesthesia-Related neuro-Toxicity in Tots' (SmartTots)" to support research on this issue. The European Society of Anaesthesiology (ESA) also initiated the project "EUROpean Safe Tots Anaesthesia Research (EUROSTAR)" to support and facilitate meetings and communication between research groups.

Several observational studies were initiated to investigate on this issue utilizing cohort data. If no significant effects of exposure to anesthesia in infancy were found by these studies, the safety of anesthetics would have been believed. However, this was not the case. Some, but not all of these, studies suggested the association between anesthesia exposure during infancy and long-term neurodevelopmental changes, although a definitive conclusion was not made because of methodological limitations common to retrospective observational studies. These studies prompted subsequent investigations with more robust tools to obtain stronger evidence on outcomes after exposure to anesthetics. Currently, several clinical studies with a prospective and/or randomized trial design are ongoing to investigate whether anesthesia is safe for young children.

2.2 Retrospective Studies

To date, the majority of findings on the neurotoxicity of anesthetics in human models have been obtained from retrospective studies, whereas findings from prospective studies have only begun to emerge in recent years. Although many studies have been conducted, an agreement in expected outcomes has yet to be established. Some studies have reported a significant association between the incidence of poor neurodevelopmental outcomes and exposure to general anesthetics during infancy, while others did not. In this section, representative retrospective studies of this topic are summarized.

2.2.1 *Retrospective Studies Without Sibling or Twin Control*

Findings from retrospective cohort studies begun to emerge from 2009. These studies used observational method taking advantage of existing birth cohort, hospital, or health register data. Despite methodological limitations, these retrospective studies have provided important clues on this topic in a short period of time.

2.2.1.1 Population-Based Cohort Study in Minnesota, USA

The population-based birth cohort study conducted by Wilder and colleagues at Mayo Clinic in the USA [5] is a landmark study that investigated the long-term neurodevelopmental effects of general anesthetics in children by using a large sample. They selected a cohort of children born between 1976 and 1982 in the five townships of Olmsted County, Minnesota. Of 5357 children, 593 children received general anesthesia before 4 years of age and the authors reviewed learning disabilities of these children available in this registry. They found that there was an increased risk of learning disability prior to 19 years of age among those with two or more instances of exposure to anesthesia, or a cumulative anesthesia duration of more than 120 min [5]. Interestingly, there was not a significant association between the incidence of learning disability and only one exposure to anesthesia.

Using the same cohort, Sprung et al. conducted another study to examine the neurodevelopmental effects of prenatal/fetal anesthetic exposure during labor and delivery [6]. In this cohort, 4823 children were delivered vaginally and 497 were delivered by a cesarean section. Among these delivered by a cesarean section, 193 received general anesthesia and 304 received regional anesthesia. No differences were found in the incidence of subsequent learning disabilities between these groups. In addition, no increased risk of subsequent learning disabilities was found among children exposed to anesthetics prior to birth.

Flick et al. performed another study using the same cohort [7]. In this study, 350 children who were exposed to anesthesia before 2 years of age were matched to 700 unexposed children based on potential confounders of learning disabilities such as sex, birth weight, health status, and gestational age. The authors observed a significantly increased risk of learning disability after multiple exposures to anesthetics, consistent with the results reported by Wilder et al. [5].

Sprung et al. also conducted another study to examine the correlation between anesthetic exposure and attention-deficit/hyperactivity disorder (ADHD) using the same cohort [8]. The authors observed that multiple exposures, but not a single exposure, were associated with an increased risk of ADHD after adjustment for confounders, consistent with the results reported by Wilder et al. [5].

2.2.1.2 Population-Based Cohort Study in New York, USA

DiMaggio and colleagues at Columbia University in the USA conducted population-based birth cohort study that examined the association between learning disabilities and exposure to general anesthetics [9]. They analyzed a cohort of children born between 1999 and 2001 from the New York Medicaid records [9]. They identified 383 children with inguinal hernia repair under 3 years of age and 5050 children without history of hernia, matched for age. The authors showed that a single exposure to anesthetics resulted in a 2.3-fold increase of risk for subsequent developmental or behavioral diagnoses.

2.2.1.3 Population-Based Cohort Study in Western Australia

Ing and colleagues at Columbia University in the USA collaborated with the Australian institutes to examine the association between exposure to anesthesia and neurodevelopmental outcomes among children born between 1989 and 1992 in the Western Australian Pregnancy Cohort [10]. Of 2608 children, 321 were exposed to anesthesia before 3 years of age, and 2287 were unexposed. The authors reviewed neurodevelopmental outcomes in language ability, cognitive function, motor skills, and behavior available in the registry. They observed that children exposed to anesthesia had a higher risk of language and cognition impairments compared to unexposed children at 10 years of age. After adjusting for demographic characteristics, the estimated hazard ratio of disability in language for children with exposure was 1.87 (95% confidence interval [CI], 1.20–2.93) and that of cognition was 1.69 (95% CI, 1.13–2.53). Conversely, motor function did not differ significantly between the exposed and unexposed groups.

2.2.1.4 Hospital-Based Cohort Study at the Academic Pediatric Hospital of the University Medical Center Utrecht, the Netherlands

Kalkman and colleagues at the University Medical Center Utrecht in the Netherlands conducted a hospital-based cohort study that examined neurobehavioral development as a function of age at the time of the first exposure to anesthesia [11]. This study analyzed a cohort of children who were operated for pediatric urological surgery between 1987 and 1995 in their hospital. A total of 243 children, up to 6 years of age, received anesthesia in this cohort. The author examined the odds ratios for a clinically deviant score as a function of age at the time of the first surgery. The adjusted odds ratio was 1.38 (95% CI, 0.59–3.22) for children under 6 months of age, 1.19 (95% CI, 0.45–3.18) for children between the ages of 6 and 12 months, and 1.20 (95% CI, 0.45–3.20) for children between the ages of 12 and 24 months. However, this was more akin to a pilot study, because the sample size was too small to yield statistically significant results.

2.2.1.5 Nationwide Cohort Study in Denmark

Hansen and colleagues at Odense University Hospital in Denmark conducted a nationwide birth cohort study that examined the association between exposure to surgery and anesthesia for inguinal hernia repair in infancy and subsequent academic performance [12]. This study selected children who underwent inguinal hernia repair under 1 year of age between 1986 and 1990 from Danish birth cohorts. The exposure group consisted of 2547 children and an age-matched control group consisted of 13,640 children. The exposed group performed more poorly than the control group before adjusting for known confounders such as gender, birth weight, and parental education. However, after adjustment for these factors, there was no statistically significant difference between the exposed and unexposed group.

Hansen and colleagues conducted another study to investigate the effects of anesthesia associated with surgery for pyloric stenosis among children under 3 months of age by using the same cohort [13]. The exposure group consisted of 779 individuals and the control group consisted of 14,665 individuals. The results were similar to those of previous study by this group [12].

Clausen et al., members of the same research group, conducted a study to investigate academic achievement of children who received anesthesia for cleft operations in infants using the same birth cohort [14]. The exposure group was consisted of 509 children and the control group of 14,677 children, which was a 5% sample of the birth cohort. Compared to controls, children with cleft lip surgery achieved higher scores of academic achievement whereas children with a cleft palate had lower scores. Children with both cleft lip and cleft palate showed lower scores on academic achievement. However, these differences were not statistically significant. Therefore the authors concluded that anesthesia was not a risk factor for neurodevelopmental impairment, although the anesthetic neurotoxicity cannot be completely excluded [14].

2.2.1.6 Nationwide Cohort Study in Taiwan

Chien and colleagues at Taipei Medical University in Taiwan conducted a nationwide birth cohort study that investigated the association between development of ASD and general anesthesia during cesarean delivery [15]. This study selected a large sample of children born between 2004 and 2007 from national data sources in Taiwan [15]. They identified 362,297 children with vaginal delivery, 161,992 children with cesarean section under regional anesthesia, and 12,384 children with cesarean section under general anesthesia. The incidences of autism per 1000 person-years was 0.77 (95% CI, 0.73–0.81), 0.92 (95% CI, 0.85–1.00), and 1.34 (95% CI, 1.06–1.69) for vaginal deliveries, cesarean section under regional anesthesia, and cesarean section under general anesthesia, respectively. Thus, the authors concluded that the risk of ASD development was associated with cesarean section under general anesthesia, contrary to the result of the study by Sprung et al. [6]. On the other hand, the risks of ASD development in neonates delivered by cesarean section under regional anesthesia and in neonates delivered virginally were not significantly different. However, there might be a bias because general anesthesia during cesarean section is predominantly used for women with pregnancy complications or emergency birth. For instance, pregnancy complications are tend to be associated with increased risk of autism.

2.2.1.7 Hospital-Based Cohort Study at the University of California San Francisco, USA

Stratmann and colleagues at the University of California San Francisco in the USA conducted a hospital-based cohort study that examined the association between anesthesia exposure during early childhood and recognition memory later in adulthood [16]. The authors retrospectively selected children aged 6–11 who received general anesthesia before 1 year of age and age- and sex-matched control subjects who did not receive anesthesia. They identified 28 children who were exposed to anesthetics in the anesthesia billing databases in 2004 at the University of California San Francisco or at the University of California Davis in the USA. The control children were selected from a registry of parents who had previously expressed interest in having their children participate in research. This selection was conducted after the start of the study as a prospective aspect of this study. The main finding was that exposure to anesthesia during infancy impaired recollection memory, although IQ was not significantly affected [16]. However, the sample size of this study was small.

2.2.1.8 Nationwide Cohort Study in Sweden

Glatz and colleagues at Kalmar County Hospital and Karolinska Institutet in Sweden conducted a nationwide cohort study that examined long-term neurodevelopmental effects of general anesthetics in children by using a large sample [17]. This study selected a cohort of children born between 1973 and 1993 in Sweden. Of 2,174,073 children, the authors identified 33,514 children who received single anesthesia before 4 years of age, 3640 with multiple anesthesia before 4 years of age, and 159,619 matched unexposed controls. The academic and cognitive performances of these children were indexed by school grades at 16 years of age and IQ test scores at 18 years of age. Children who received single anesthesia before 4 years of age showed a statistically significant lower school grades and IQ test scores compared with controls, although the differences were small. The magnitude of the difference was the same after multiple exposures. Interestingly, these differences were markedly less than the differences associated with sex, maternal educational level, or month of birth during the same year. Thus, the authors stated that many other factors were far more important than anesthesia exposure in children regarding the long-term neurodevelopmental effects [17].

2.2.2 *Retrospective Studies with Sibling or Twin Control*

An important weakness of the above-mentioned retrospective studies is the inability to dissociate the effects of general anesthesia from the many potentially confounding factors. Twin and sibling study designs are attractive tools, which are commonly utilized in psychiatric studies since a large number of potential confounders are controlled within each twin and sibling pair. For instance, environmental and genetic differences in individuals can be addressed by these study designs. In particular, the environmental bias of parental education and socioeconomic status are relevant and important confounding factors in neurocognitive studies [24]. Furthermore, these study designs would address many confounders that might be unmeasured in traditional cohort studies. Several researchers have conducted studies by using these designs to dissociate the effects of general anesthesia from the many potentially confounding factors.

2.2.2.1 Nationwide Twin Cohort Study in the Netherlands

Bartels and colleagues at VU University in the Netherlands conducted a nationwide twin birth cohort study that investigated the association between anesthesia exposure and school performance among children [18]. This study selected monozygotic twin pairs born between 1986 and 1995 from the Young Netherlands Twin Registry. The cohort comprised 1143 monozygotic twin pairs. The authors reviewed educational achievement and cognitive problems evaluated by standardized test scores and teacher ratings at 12 years of age available in this registry. There was a correlation between the incidence of learning disabilities and anesthesia exposure among children under the age of 3 years. However, in discordant twin pairs (where one twin was exposed to anesthesia and the other was not), there was no difference between twins. Therefore the authors concluded that there was no relationship between exposure to anesthesia and cognitive performance later in life. However, the Mayo Clinic group et al. criticized this conclusion, citing an inaccurate assessment of educational achievement [19].

2.2.2.2 Population-Based Sibling Cohort Study in New York, USA

DiMaggio and colleagues at Columbia University in the USA conducted a population-based sibling cohort study that investigated the association between the number of anesthesia exposures and the risk of developmental or behavioral impairment. This study selected siblings born between 1999 and 2005 from the New York Medicaid records [20]. Of 10,450 siblings, 304 children underwent surgery when they were younger than 3 years of age and 10,146 children did not. After adjusting for sex and history of birth-related medical complications, as well as clustering by sibling status, the estimated hazard ratio for developmental or behavioral disorders was 1.1 (95% CI, 0.8–1.4) for a single exposure to anesthetics, 2.9 (95% CI, 2.5–3.1) for two exposures, and 4.0 (95% CI, 3.5–4.5) for more than two exposures.

2.2.2.3 Population-Based Sibling Case-Control Study in Puerto Rico

Creagh and colleagues at the University of Puerto Rico in Puerto Rico conducted a population-based sibling case-control study that investigated the association between anesthesia exposures and ASD. This study selected 262 children with ASD and 253 without ASD (sibling of children with ASD) born in Puerto Rico [21]. They assessed variables including demographics, diagnosis, severity of ASD, exposure to anesthesia, and age at exposure among sibling pairs. Of the 262 patients with ASD, 99 had exposure to anesthetics prior to their diagnosis. Of the 253 individuals without ASD, 110 had been exposed to anesthesia. Therefore, the authors concluded that exposure to anesthesia in children did not increase the probability of developing ASD.

2.2.3 *Limitation of Retrospective Studies*

Although the above-mentioned studies provide important insights into this topic, these studies have a number of limitations which impose caution in interpreting results. Some of these limitations are inherently related to the nature of a retrospective cohort study. Limitations of these studies are reviewed in this section.

2.2.3.1 Characteristics of Anesthetics Used

In many of the retrospective cohort studies mentioned above, children were exposed to general anesthesia during the late 1970s and early 1980s. As pointed out by some investigators, general anesthetics used during this period were different from those in use today (for review see [22, 23]). In the study by Wilder et al. [5], the most frequently used combination of anesthetics was nitrous oxide (88.1%) and halothane (87.5%). Kalkman et al. [11] also reported that halothane was commonly used in their data. Since the early 1980s, however, halothane was no longer a part of common clinical applications, and the use of nitrous oxide had declined. Therefore, the anesthetic characteristics were significantly different from that currently in use in the field of anesthesiology. In this relation, the study by DiMaggio et al. [8] lacked precise information on anesthetic exposure and specific drugs used, although the duration, cumulative doses, and specific anesthetics used likely affect neurodevelopmental outcomes [24, 25].

2.2.3.2 Lack of Standardization in Outcome Measures

Some studies lacked standardization of outcome measures due to poorly defined outcome endpoints. For instance, the outcome of "learning disability" used in the study by Wilder et al. [5] was heterogeneous, meaning that three different types of indexes "reading, written language, and math disabilities" were combined into a single outcome measure. Therefore "learning disability" as defined by this study was a categorical determination and not a specific neuropsychological outcome (for review see [23]). The International Classification of Disease 9th Revision (ICD-9) diagnostic codes used in the study by DiMaggio et al. [9] were possibly also limited, because these codes may be subject to variations in local coding practices and conventions as well as misclassification from diagnostic coding (for review see [23]). The academic achievement scores in the study by Bartels et al. [17] were possibly also limited because these scores reported by teachers may be influenced by many biases (for review see [21]).

2.2.3.3 Other Confounding Factors

There are a large number of potential confounders to adjust in this issue. Furthermore, many confounders may remain unknown. One of the most important confounders is that children who receive anesthesia do so to undergo a surgical or an imaging procedure, so interpretation of the results should be cautious. The outcomes are inevitably associated with the underlying pathology that necessitated the use of anesthesia and surgery. In addition, other comorbidities such as surgical procedures might likewise contribute to neurodevelopmental outcomes. Surgical procedures may cause trauma including inflammatory responses, hemodynamic changes, and hypothermia, which are all secondary to the surgical procedure itself.

2.2.4 Meta-Analysis

In this section, meta-analysis of some retrospective studies is reviewed.

2.2.4.1 Meta-Analysis of Retrospective Studies

Wang and colleagues completed a meta-analysis of seven retrospective studies mentioned above (published between January 1, 2000, and February 1, 2013) [4, 8–12, 18] to summarize the association between anesthesia exposure during early childhood and behavioral outcomes later in life [26]. The authors estimated the synthesized hazard ratio to be 1.25 (95% CI, 1.13–1.38, $P < 0.001$) for the association of anesthesia exposure under 4 years of age and neurodevelopmental impairments.

The authors also showed that the multiple exposure to anesthesia was a risk factor for neurodevelopmental impairment; the hazard ratio among those children was 1.75 (95% CI, 1.31–2.33, $P < 0.001$).

2.3 Prospective Studies

The results of some above-mentioned retrospective studies could not indicate the association between anesthesia exposure during infancy and long-term neurodevelopmental changes definitively. Thus, in the next step, stronger evidence using more powerful tools is needed. In a prospective trial, standardization of outcome measures can be definitively validated prior to the start of the study. In this section, several prospective studies are reviewed.

2.3.1 Semi-prospective Studies

In several studies, the outcome measures are definitively developed before any subjects returned for follow-up assessments, although subjects were retrospectively selected. Thus, these studies are semi-prospective or ambidirectional, meaning the use of a prospective assessment for a retrospective cohort.

2.3.1.1 The PANDA (Pediatric Anesthesia Neurodevelopment Assessment) Study

The PANDA study is a nationwide multicenter sibling-controlled cohort study with ambidirectional design, which investigates the long-term effects of anesthesia on cognitive functions. This study is conducted by the PANDA Network that is based at Columbia University and involves eight study sites in the USA. This study assesses the long-term effects of anesthesia on global cognitive function (IQ) as the primary outcome. This study identified a cohort of retrospectively obtained 500 sibling pairs discordant for a single exposure to anesthesia prior to 36 months of age for elective inguinal hernia repair surgery. The follow-up period is 15 years with neurodevelopmental and cognitive assessments at 8 and 15 years of age.

Although the PANDA study is not completed, two interim reports were published to date. In 2012, the authors reported on the results of a small pilot study comparing 28 sibling pairs at 6–11 years of age, which was performed to confirm the feasibility of the study design [27]. The pilot data did not show significant differences in global cognitive function between the groups. In 2016, the authors reported on the result of a study comparing 105 sibling pairs at 10 years of age [28]. There was no statistically significant differences in IQ scores between the groups.

2.3.1.2 The MASK (Mayo Anesthesia Safety in Kids) Study

The MASK study is a population-based birth cohort study with ambidirectional design, which investigates whether exposure of children to anesthesia prior to age 3 is associated with neurodevelopmental abnormalities. The MASK study is conducted by Mayo Clinic and National Center for Toxicological Research in the USA. This study identified a cohort of all children born in Olmsted County, Minnesota, between the years 1994 and 2007, who are currently local residents. This study selected children with multiple, single, and no anesthesia exposure prior to the age of 3 years and assesses neuropsychological traits of these children by using neurocognitive test batteries that were definitively developed prior to the start of the study [29]. This study is ongoing.

2.3.2 *Prospective Randomized Study*

A randomized controlled trial is an attractive design that can avoid many of the limitations that plague previous retrospective cohort studies. This design can address many of the confounding factors and even unknown confounding factors which cannot be excluded by matching to controls [30]. However, it is not reasonable to administer general anesthetics to healthy children for ethical reasons. It is also not possible to perform surgery on children without anesthesia. Therefore, a placebo-controlled randomized clinical trial is seldom feasible. However, one study has been conducted addressing these difficulties.

2.3.2.1 The GAS (General Anesthesia and Spinal) Study

The GAS study is an international multicenter cohort study with randomized controlled design, which examines the effect of general anesthesia in infancy on neurodevelopmental outcome. The GAS study is conducted by the GAS consortium, which is based at the Boston Children's Hospital in the USA and the Royal Children's Hospital Melbourne in Australia and includes 28 hospitals in Australia, Italy, the USA, the UK, Canada, the Netherlands, and New Zealand. This study selected 772 infants who received inguinal hernia repair under the postmenstrual age of 60 weeks at the time of surgery. Participants were randomly assigned to receive either general or regional anesthesia. The general anesthesia group received sevoflurane one time with duration less than 1 h and comprised 359 children. The regional anesthesia group comprised 363 children. This study analyzes neurodevelopmental outcomes by neurodevelopment and intelligence testing. The follow-up period will be 5 years with assessments at 2 and 5 years of age. This is the first and thus far only randomized clinical study of this topic.

Although the GAS study is not completed, one interim report was published. In 2015, the evaluation of neurodevelopmental outcomes at 2 years of age was published by Davidson et al. [31]. The authors did not find significant differences in neurodevelopmental outcomes between the groups. However, the authors noted a limitation in the sensitivity of the developmental assessment: "at 2 years of age, it is difficult to accurately diagnose the presence of disorders such as autism spectrum disorder" [31]. Thus, these results did not provide the definitive evidence in outcomes and the final analyses at 5 years of age are needed to provide the conclusion.

2.3.3 Limitations of Prospective and Randomized Studies

Although prospective and randomized study design will provide robust evidence and important information, they have some limitations. Prospective studies take too much time to complete because the follow-up period between anesthesia exposure and assessment will be extremely long. Thus, the definitive conclusion has not yet been made.

In the GAS study, participants were limited to those exposed to anesthesia only at one time. If the GAS study does not find that a brief or single exposure to anesthesia causes adverse outcomes, they cannot rule out the possibility that longer or multiple exposures might cause changes in neurodevelopmental outcomes. It would be very difficult to design a randomized trial to evaluate the possibility that multiple exposures may be necessary to produce adverse neurodevelopmental outcomes in humans [32]. Furthermore, it is not possible to know "whether one exposure to anesthesia, which might not have consequences, will eventually become an element of several exposures to anesthesia, which might" [32]. In the GAS study, the mean duration of general anesthesia was 54 min in order to match that of the spinal anesthesia. As noted by the authors themselves [30], this exposure duration was relatively brief because most animal studies suggest that usually 2 or 3 h is needed to induce changes in neurodevelopmental outcomes.

2.4 Prevention and Treatment

If children undergo surgery, exposure to anesthetics is unavoidable in many cases because there is no substitute. Development of methods to prevent potential neurotoxicity of anesthetics in infants has been conducted for the safety of pediatric anesthesia prior to making a comprehensive conclusion regarding the neurotoxicity in humans. Although most of these studies are not completed, a few studies are reviewed in this section.

2.4.1 *Change in Anesthesia Practice?*

At present, a comprehensive conclusion is not possible from the human studies mentioned above. It is therefore difficult to make any recommendations for specific practice guidelines or changes to pediatric anesthesia.

Many retrospective cohort studies mentioned above have assessed children who received anesthesia prior to 3 years of age. However, there is no date for any safe age cutoff. The safe age cutoff cannot be extrapolated from animal studies because of interspecies differences in brain development.

2.4.2 *Dexmedetomidine-Based Anesthesia*

An animal study reported that dexmedetomidine may be beneficial in avoiding the deleterious effects of general anesthesia on neurodevelopment [33]. Bong and colleagues at the KK Women's and Children's Hospital in Singapore investigated the feasibility of dexmedetomidine-based anesthesia in place of general anesthetics among infants [34]. The authors retrospectively reviewed a case series of 50 infants who received dexmedetomidine sedation with caudal anesthesia instead of general anesthesia for inguinal hernia repair. The authors found that no patient developed significant bradycardia or required intubation. Thus, they concluded that this method may be a feasible alternative. However, a long-term follow-up to assess neurodevelopmental outcomes has not been conducted.

Similar to the study by Bong et al. [34], the T REX pilot study based at the Murdoch Children's Research Institute in Australia, investigated the feasibility of dexmedetomidine-based anesthesia for lower limb, urologic, or lower abdominal procedures in infants. This study used dexmedetomidine and an opioid (remifentanil) combined with caudal analgesia. The outcomes were the need for intervention for mild anesthesia, intervention for hemodynamic changes, and rate of abandoning the protocol. This study has been completed but the results remain yet to be seen.

References

1. Levy D (1945) Psychic trauma of operations in children and a note on combat neurosis. Am J Dis Child 69:7–25
2. Jevtovic-Todorovic V, Hartman RE, Izumi Y, Benshoff ND, Dikranian K, Zorumski CF, Olney JW, Wozniak DF (2003) Early exposure to common anesthetic agents causes widespread neurodegeneration in the developing rat brain and persistent learning deficits. J Neurosci Off J Soc Neurosci 23(3):876–882
3. Satomoto M, Satoh Y, Terui K, Miyao H, Takishima K, Ito M, Imaki J (2009) Neonatal exposure to sevoflurane induces abnormal social behaviors and deficits in fear conditioning in mice. Anesthesiology 110(3):628–637. doi:10.1097/ALN.0b013e3181974fa2

4. DeFrances CJ, Cullen KA, Kozak LJ (2007) National Hospital Discharge Survey: 2005 annual summary with detailed diagnosis and procedure data. Vit Health Stat Series 13, Data from the National Health Survey (165):1–209
5. Wilder RT, Flick RP, Sprung J, Katusic SK, Barbaresi WJ, Mickelson C, Gleich SJ, Schroeder DR, Weaver AL, Warner DO (2009) Early exposure to anesthesia and learning disabilities in a population-based birth cohort. Anesthesiology 110(4):796–804. doi:10.1097/01.anes.0000344728.34332.5d
6. Sprung J, Flick RP, Wilder RT, Katusic SK, Pike TL, Dingli M, Gleich SJ, Schroeder DR, Barbaresi WJ, Hanson AC, Warner DO (2009) Anesthesia for cesarean delivery and learning disabilities in a population-based birth cohort. Anesthesiology 111(2):302–310. doi:10.1097/ALN.0b013e3181adf481
7. Flick RP, Katusic SK, Colligan RC, Wilder RT, Voigt RG, Olson MD, Sprung J, Weaver AL, Schroeder DR, Warner DO (2011) Cognitive and behavioral outcomes after early exposure to anesthesia and surgery. Pediatrics 128(5):e1053–e1061. doi:10.1542/peds.2011-0351
8. Sprung J, Flick RP, Katusic SK, Colligan RC, Barbaresi WJ, Bojanic K, Welch TL, Olson MD, Hanson AC, Schroeder DR, Wilder RT, Warner DO (2012) Attention-deficit/hyperactivity disorder after early exposure to procedures requiring general anesthesia. Mayo Clin Proc 87(2):120–129. doi:10.1016/j.mayocp.2011.11.008
9. DiMaggio C, Sun LS, Kakavouli A, Byrne MW, Li G (2009) A retrospective cohort study of the association of anesthesia and hernia repair surgery with behavioral and developmental disorders in young children. J Neurosurg Anesthesiol 21(4):286–291. doi:10.1097/ANA.0b013e3181a71f11
10. Ing C, DiMaggio C, Whitehouse A, Hegarty MK, Brady J, von Ungern-Sternberg BS, Davidson A, Wood AJ, Li G, Sun LS (2012) Long-term differences in language and cognitive function after childhood exposure to anesthesia. Pediatrics 130(3):e476–e485. doi:10.1542/peds.2011-3822
11. Kalkman CJ, Peelen L, Moons KG, Veenhuizen M, Bruens M, Sinnema G, de Jong TP (2009) Behavior and development in children and age at the time of first anesthetic exposure. Anesthesiology 110(4):805–812. doi:10.1097/ALN.0b013e31819c7124
12. Hansen TG, Pedersen JK, Henneberg SW, Pedersen DA, Murray JC, Morton NS, Christensen K (2011) Academic performance in adolescence after inguinal hernia repair in infancy: a nationwide cohort study. Anesthesiology 114(5):1076–1085. doi:10.1097/ALN.0b013e31820e77a0
13. Hansen TG, Pedersen JK, Henneberg SW, Morton NS, Christensen K (2013) Educational outcome in adolescence following pyloric stenosis repair before 3 months of age: a nationwide cohort study. Paediatr Anaesth 23(10):883–890. doi:10.1111/pan.12225
14. Clausen NG, Pedersen DA, Pedersen JK, Moller SE, Grosen D, Wehby GL, Christensen K, Hansen TG (2016) Oral clefts and academic performance in adolescence: the impact of anesthesia-related neurotoxicity, timing of surgery, and type of oral clefts. Cleft Palate Craniofac J. doi:10.1597/15-185
15. Chien LN, Lin HC, Shao YH, Chiou ST, Chiou HY (2015) Risk of autism associated with general anesthesia during cesarean delivery: a population-based birth-cohort analysis. J Autism Dev Disord 45(4):932–942. doi:10.1007/s10803-014-2247-y
16. Stratmann G, Lee J, Sall JW, Lee BH, Alvi RS, Shih J, Rowe AM, Ramage TM, Chang FL, Alexander TG, Lempert DK, Lin N, Siu KH, Elphick SA, Wong A, Schnair CI, Vu AF, Chan JT, Zai H, Wong MK, Anthony AM, Barbour KC, Ben-Tzur D, Kazarian NE, Lee JY, Shen JR, Liu E, Behniwal GS, Lammers CR, Quinones Z, Aggarwal A, Cedars E, Yonelinas AP, Ghetti S (2014) Effect of general anesthesia in infancy on long-term recognition memory in humans and rats. Neuropsychopharmacology 39(10):2275–2287. doi:10.1038/npp.2014.134
17. Glatz P, Sandin RH, Pedersen NL, Bonamy AK, Eriksson LI, Granath F (2017) Association of anesthesia and surgery during childhood with long-term academic performance. JAMA Pediatr 171(1):e163470. doi:10.1001/jamapediatrics.2016.3470
18. Bartels M, Althoff RR, Boomsma DI (2009) Anesthesia and cognitive performance in children: no evidence for a causal relationship. Twin Res Hum Genet 12(3):246–253. doi:10.1375/twin.12.3.246

19. Flick RP, Wilder RT, Sprung J, Katusic SK, Voigt R, Colligan R, Schroeder DR, Weaver AL, Warner DO (2009) Anesthesia and cognitive performance in children: no evidence for a causal relationship. Are the conclusions justified by the data? Response to Bartels et al., 2009. Twin Res Hum Genet 12(6):611–612 . doi:10.1375/twin.12.6.611discussion 613–614
20. DiMaggio C, Sun LS, Li G (2011) Early childhood exposure to anesthesia and risk of developmental and behavioral disorders in a sibling birth cohort. Anesth Analg 113(5):1143–1151. doi:10.1213/ANE.0b013e3182147f42
21. Creagh O, Torres H, Rivera K, Morales-Franqui M, Altieri-Acevedo G, Warner D (2015) Previous exposure to anesthesia and autism spectrum disorder (ASD): a Puerto Rican Population-Based Sibling Cohort Study. Bol Asoc Med P R 107(3):29–37
22. Sinner B, Becke K, Engelhard K (2014) General anaesthetics and the developing brain: an overview. Anaesthesia 69(9):1009–1022. doi:10.1111/anae.12637
23. Sun L (2010) Early childhood general anaesthesia exposure and neurocognitive development. Br J Anaesth 105(Suppl 1):i61–i68. doi:10.1093/bja/aeq302
24. Kodama M, Satoh Y, Otsubo Y, Araki Y, Yonamine R, Masui K, Kazama T (2011) Neonatal desflurane exposure induces more robust neuroapoptosis than do isoflurane and sevoflurane and impairs working memory. Anesthesiology 115(5):979–991. doi:10.1097/ALN.0b013e318234228b
25. Liang G, Ward C, Peng J, Zhao Y, Huang B, Wei H (2010) Isoflurane causes greater neurodegeneration than an equivalent exposure of sevoflurane in the developing brain of neonatal mice. Anesthesiology 112(6):1325–1334. doi:10.1097/ALN.0b013e3181d94da5
26. Wang X, Xu Z, Miao CH (2014) Current clinical evidence on the effect of general anesthesia on neurodevelopment in children: an updated systematic review with meta-regression. PLoS One 9(1):e85760. doi:10.1371/journal.pone.0085760
27. Sun LS, Li G, DiMaggio CJ, Byrne MW, Ing C, Miller TL, Bellinger DC, Han S, McGowan FX (2012) Feasibility and pilot study of the Pediatric Anesthesia NeuroDevelopment Assessment (PANDA) project. J Neurosurg Anesthesiol 24(4):382–388. doi:10.1097/ANA.0b013e31826a0371
28. Sun LS, Li G, Miller TL, Salorio C, Byrne MW, Bellinger DC, Ing C, Park R, Radcliffe J, Hays SR, DiMaggio CJ, Cooper TJ, Rauh V, Maxwell LG, Youn A, McGowan FX (2016) Association between a single general anesthesia exposure before age 36 months and neurocognitive outcomes in later childhood. JAMA 315(21):2312–2320. doi:10.1001/jama.2016.6967
29. Gleich SJ, Flick R, Hu D, Zaccariello MJ, Colligan RC, Katusic SK, Schroeder DR, Hanson A, Buenvenida S, Wilder RT, Sprung J, Voigt RG, Paule MG, Chelonis JJ, Warner DO (2015) Neurodevelopment of children exposed to anesthesia: design of the Mayo Anesthesia Safety in Kids (MASK) study. Contemp Clin Trials 41:45–54. doi:10.1016/j.cct.2014.12.020
30. Davidson AJ, McCann ME, Morton NS, Myles PS (2008) Anesthesia and outcome after neonatal surgery: the role for randomized trials. Anesthesiology 109(6):941–944. doi:10.1097/ALN.0b013e31818e3f79
31. Davidson AJ, Disma N, de Graaff JC, Withington DE, Dorris L, Bell G, Stargatt R, Bellinger DC, Schuster T, Arnup SJ, Hardy P, Hunt RW, Takagi MJ, Giribaldi G, Hartmann PL, Salvo I, Morton NS, von Ungern Sternberg BS, Locatelli BG, Wilton N, Lynn A, Thomas JJ, Polaner D, Bagshaw O, Szmuk P, Absalom AR, Frawley G, Berde C, Ormond GD, Marmor J, McCann ME, GAS consortium (2016) Neurodevelopmental outcome at 2 years of age after general anaesthesia and awake-regional anaesthesia in infancy (GAS): an international multicentre, randomised controlled trial. Lancet 387(10015):239–250. doi:10.1016/S0140-6736(15)00608-X
32. Warner DO, Flick RP (2016) Anaesthetics, infants, and neurodevelopment: case closed? Lancet 387(10015):202–204. doi:10.1016/S0140-6736(15)00669-8
33. Sanders RD, Xu J, Shu Y, Januszewski A, Halder S, Fidalgo A, Sun P, Hossain M, Ma D, Maze M (2009) Dexmedetomidine attenuates isoflurane-induced neurocognitive impairment in neonatal rats. Anesthesiology 110(5):1077–1085. doi:10.1097/ALN.0b013e31819daedd
34. Bong CL, Yeo AS, Fabila T, Tan JS (2016) A pilot study of dexmedetomidine sedation and caudal anesthesia for inguinal hernia repair in infants. Paediatr Anaesth. doi:10.1111/pan.12907

Chapter 3
Implications for Pediatric Anesthesia

Koichi Yuki, Yasushi Mio, and Shoichi Uezono

Abstract Preclinical studies have shown that volatile and intravenous anesthetics increase neuroapoptosis in neonatal rodents and monkeys. These results raise concerns regarding the use of anesthetics in young children. Retrospective reports suggest an association between multiple surgeries under anesthesia at infancy and subsequent learning disabilities. Anesthesia is a requisite component of surgeries and procedures, and as anesthesia providers, it is important that we understand what is known about the risks of anesthesia in the developing brain. The aim of this chapter is to review the literature with respect to anesthesia-related neurotoxicity in neonatal animals and young children.

Keywords Anesthetics • Apoptosis • Neurotoxicity • Pediatrics

3.1 Introduction

There has been a growing concern regarding the potential of anesthetics to cause neurotoxicity in children. A landmark study by Ikonomidou and colleagues in 1999 suggested that *N*-methyl-D-aspartic acid (NMDA) antagonists increase apoptosis in the neonatal rat brain up to postnatal day 14 (P14) [1]. The same group reported in 2000 that γ-aminobutyric acid (GABA) receptor agonists also increase apoptosis in the neonatal rat brain [2]. Although the mechanisms of action of some anesthetics are yet to be determined, NMDA and $GABA_A$ receptors are believed to be prime targets for anesthesia in the central nervous system (Table 3.1). Investigators have since conducted studies to delineate if anesthetics can indeed result in neurotoxicity.

K. Yuki, M.D.
Cardiac Anesthesia Division, Department of Anesthesiology, Perioperative and Pain Medicine, Boston Children's Hospital, Boston, MA, USA

Y. Mio, M.D. • S. Uezono, M.D. (✉)
Department of Anesthesia, Jikei University,
3-25-8 Nishishimbashi, Minato-ku, Tokyo 105-0003, Japan
e-mail: uezono@jikei.ac.jp

Y. Morimoto (ed.), *Anesthesia and Neurotoxicity*,
DOI 10.1007/978-4-431-55624-4_3

Table 3.1 Anesthetics that interact with NMDA and $GABA_A$ receptors

NMDA receptor	$GABA_A$ receptor
Ketamine	Midazolam
Nitrous oxide	Propofol
Xenon	Etomidate
	Thiopental
	Isoflurane
	Sevoflurane

GABA γ-aminobutyric acid, *NMDA* *N*-methyl-D-aspartic acid

A 2003 study by Jevtovic-Todorovic and colleagues showed that early exposure to common anesthetic agents (a combination of midazolam, isoflurane, and nitrous oxide) induces widespread apoptosis in the neonatal rat brain, along with subsequent functional impairments [3]. That study was alarming enough to facilitate worldwide anesthesia neurotoxicity research. In 2007, the US Food and Drug Administration (FDA) announced that anesthesia drugs pose a risk of potential neurotoxicity in pediatric patients, though "there are not adequate data to extrapolate the animal findings to humans." The FDA also collaborated with the International Anesthesia Research Society to initiate SmartTots (Strategies for Mitigating Anesthesia-Related neuroToxicity in Tots). A recently published editorial in *The New England Journal of Medicine* stated, "while we await clinical studies that can definitely determine whether anesthetics cause injury in humans, surgeons and anesthesiologists and parents should consider carefully how urgently surgery is needed, particularly under 3 years of age" [4]. On the basis of that article, *The New York Times* posted an article titled Researchers Warn on Anesthesia, Unsure of Risk to Children. As anesthesia providers for the pediatric population, it is imperative for us to understand what is known and what is unknown in order to provide the best care and information possible for patients and families and also for other medical professionals. The purpose of this review is to describe the state of the art with respect to anesthesia-related neurotoxicity in young children. Of note, anesthetics are known to provide anti-inflammatory effects and to offer neuroprotective effects in certain scenarios [5]. However, it is beyond the scope of this review to go into depth on the relation and balance between neuroprotective and neurotoxic effects of anesthetics.

3.2 Brain Development and Apoptosis

3.2.1 Neurodevelopment

The brain undergoes several generalized steps to become fully mature (Fig. 3.1). Neurulation results in the formation of the neural plate from the ectoderm and transforms the neural plate into the neural tube. Neural proliferation and migration follow to create the brain structure. Although the formation of connections between

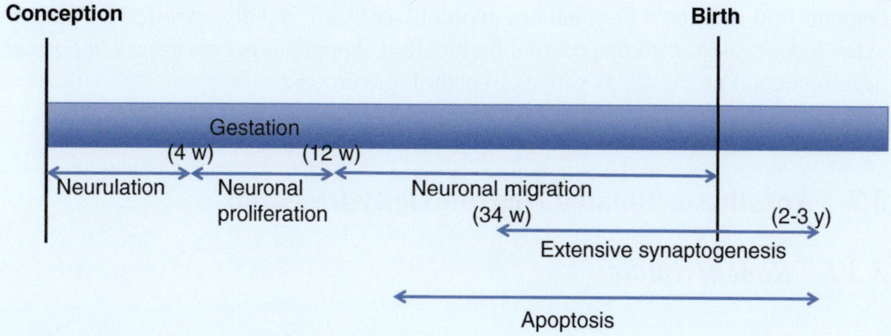

Fig. 3.1 Brain and neuronal development

neurons (synapses) is a process that lasts throughout life, an explosive formation of synapses in the central nervous system (termed "exuberant synaptogenesis") occurs in humans from the last trimester of pregnancy to the first 2–3 years of life. During this time, apoptosis, a form of programmed cell death, controls the numbers of neurons and synapses, eliminating unnecessary neurons and synapse formation. This is termed "pruning." Up to 50% of neurons are eliminated during this process. As such, it is recognized that apoptosis is a normal part of brain development.

Various mediators are critical for brain development. Glutamate is an excitatory neurotransmitter that binds to glutamate receptors, including NMDA receptors, involved in neurogenesis [6]. GABA is also a critical neurotransmitter. In the developing brain, GABA receptors are excitatory, leading to depolarization of the cell membrane as a result of a high intracellular chloride ion concentration. However, the intracellular chloride concentration decreases as the brain develops, and GABA receptors shift from excitatory to inhibitory in nature [7]. In addition, brain-derived neurotrophic factor (BDNF) regulates the differentiation of progenitor cells. It is reasonable to expect that any stimulus that alters the milieu of these mediators can affect the process of brain development.

3.2.2 Apoptosis

Apoptosis occurs via the action of cysteine proteases, termed caspases, which degrade cellular constituents. Apoptosis is largely categorized into two pathways, the extrinsic (death receptor) pathway and the intrinsic (mitochondrial) pathway. In the extrinsic pathway, various mediators activate death receptors, such as tumor necrosis factor (TNF) receptors and FAS receptors, and trigger activation of caspase 8. In the intrinsic pathway, various stimulants, including radiation, nutrition deprivation, and hypoxia, change the inner mitochondrial membrane potential and permeabilize the mitochondria, releasing cytochrome c into the cytosol. This leads to the activation of caspase 9. In both pathways, caspase 3 is subsequently activated, and DNA fragmentation follows. Different from necrosis, which releases cellular contents and induces inflammation, apoptotic cells are rapidly engulfed by phagocytes and are silent with respect to inflammation. Apoptosis occurs as part of normal developmental processes as well as in pathologic processes.

3.3 Anesthesia-Related Neurotoxicity Research

3.3.1 Rodent Studies

Rodent studies, particularly rat studies, have been the mainstay of anesthesia-related neurotoxicity research. The impact of different anesthetics on the developing brain has been assessed histologically as well as functionally. Histologic assessments largely evaluate the degree and location of apoptotic cells, whereas functional assessments involve motor function and memory. Understanding reported study designs and results is critical in applying translation to clinical practice. The purpose of this chapter is to review the available literature on this matter.

Volatile anesthetics have been popular since the development of ether anesthesia in 1848. Isoflurane, sevoflurane, and desflurane are ether-based volatile anesthetics popular in clinical practice. Nitrous oxide is a non-ether-based volatile anesthetic that has long been in use. The 2003 study by Jevtovic-Todorovic and colleagues tested midazolam (3–9 mg/kg), 0.75–1.5% isoflurane for 6 h, and 50–150% nitrous oxide for 6 h (hyperbaric conditions were used for 150% nitrous oxide), alone or in combination, in P7 rat pups [3]. Isoflurane alone induced significant apoptotic neurodegeneration in a dose-dependent manner, whereas rats treated with midazolam or nitrous oxide alone showed no significant changes compared to control rats. The combination of midazolam or nitrous oxide, or both, with isoflurane substantially increased apoptosis, particularly in the hippocampus and neocortex, compared to isoflurane alone. Combination of the three caused persistent memory and learning impairments at P131, raising concern regarding the use of anesthetics in young children. The same group studied the mechanism(s) underlying this pathologic neuroapoptosis and reported that these anesthetics induced apoptosis via both the intrinsic and extrinsic pathways, showing increased activation of caspase 9 and caspase 8, respectively (Fig. 3.2) [8]. However, the apoptotic inducers in each pathway were not explored.

Head and colleagues reported that apoptosis occurs via inhibition of tissue plasminogen activator (tPA) release from presynaptic vesicles [9]. Pro-BDNF is cleaved by plasmin, cleaved product of plasminogen by tPA, to mature BDNF(m-BDNF), which binds to tropomyosin receptor kinase B (TrkB) receptors to enhance neuronal survival and stabilize synapses. If uncleaved due to inhibition of tPA, pro-BDNF binds to neurotrophic receptor $p75^{NTR}$, and induces neuronal apoptosis and hinders synaptogenesis. Head et al. suggested that the reduction of neuronal activity by isoflurane attenuates the release of tPA, and therefore plasmin, resulting in the dominance of pro-BDNF population over m-BDNF [9]. The relation between increased

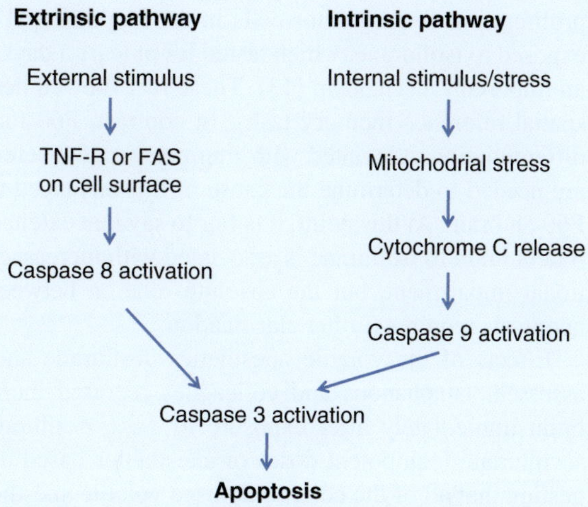

Fig. 3.2 Apoptosis pathway

pro-BDNF and caspase activation was not described in their study, but it likely involves the intrinsic pathway.

Wu and colleagues reported that isoflurane directly induces proinflammatory cytokine production (TNF-α, interleukin [IL]-1β, and IL-6) in neurons [10], and this may be in part responsible for apoptosis via the extrinsic pathway. The above studies strongly support the concept of volatile anesthesia-induced neuroapoptosis and subsequent functional impairment.

Loepke and colleagues exposed P7 rats to 1.5% isoflurane for 6 h [11]. They also found histologic evidence of apoptosis in the brain immediately after isoflurane exposure. Interestingly, they did not observe a significant reduction in adult neuronal density or functional deficits in spontaneous locomotion, spatial learning, or memory, implying that neuroapoptosis may be transient after exposure. Stratmann and colleagues examined the effect of isoflurane (1 minimum alveolar concentration [MAC]) for 1, 2, or 4 h in P7 rats [12]. Because isoflurane inhalation causes hypercarbia, they also included a group exposed to CO_2 for 4 h. They found significant neuronal apoptosis in the groups exposed to isoflurane for 2 or 4 h and in the group exposed to CO_2 for 4 h, soon after exposure. Both isoflurane and CO_2 induced significant apoptosis in the thalamus, suggesting that some of the apoptosis occurring after isoflurane exposure might be due to hypercarbia. Functional tests performed 8 weeks after exposure revealed that only the 4-h isoflurane group developed impaired spatial reference memory and spatial working memory, whereas the CO_2 group showed improvements in those parameters. On the basis of this finding, the authors concluded that isoflurane-induced cell death soon after exposure may not guarantee subsequent neurocognitive dysfunction, raising the question of whether anesthesia-related apoptosis in the developing brain is the actual culprit responsible for cognitive deficits observed after anesthesia. Whatever the underlying mechanism, this study reinforced the idea that exposure of the developing brain to isoflurane for at least 4 h impairs neurologic function in rodents. The same group reported decreased proliferation of progenitor cells in the hippocampal dentate gyrus in P7 rat brain exposed to isoflurane, which lasted for at least 5 days, suggesting that this might be an important mechanism [13]. These rats showed deficits in fear conditioning and spatial reference memory tasks. In contrast, P60 rats showed increased neuronal differentiation associated with improved spatial reference memory. Future studies are needed to determine the cause of this enhanced neuronal differentiation in the P60 rat brain. At this point, it is fair to say that extended exposure of the developing rodent brain to isoflurane is associated with increased neuronal apoptosis and functional impairment, but the absolute relation between functional impairment and apoptosis requires further clarification.

Effects of the volatile anesthetics desflurane and sevoflurane have also been assessed. Istaphanous and colleagues reported increased apoptosis in P7/P8 rat brain immediately after exposure to 7.3% desflurane, 1.6% isoflurane, or 3.2% sevoflurane (equipotent doses of anesthetics based on tail clamping) for 6 h, suggesting that all of the commonly used volatile anesthetics can induce neurotoxicity [14]. However, they did not report functional consequences. Overall, all of the currently used ether-based volatile anesthetics induce significant neuroapoptosis during the period of synaptogenesis in the rodent brain. However, the presence of apoptosis in the brain soon after anesthetic exposure does not necessarily guarantee functional impairment, and further studies are needed to determine if sevoflurane or desflurane causes functional impairment.

Most studies have focused on the location and degree of apoptosis in the developing brain; however, it is also critical to understand the effect of anesthetics on synapse formation. The study by Head et al. showed that isoflurane exposure decreases dendritic filopodial spines in P7 rat brain [9]. This may lead to impaired synaptogenesis and may serve as an additional mechanism of anesthesia-induced neurotoxicity. Similarly, Briner and colleagues studied P16 rats, which are in the developmental stage characterized by intense synaptogenesis in the cerebral cortex [15]. Rats were exposed to 1.5% isoflurane, 2.5% sevoflurane, or 7% desflurane for 30, 60, or 120 min. In contrast to the study by Head et al. [9], all of the volatile anesthetics tested increased dendrite density. In this age group, volatile anesthetics induced no significant neuroapoptosis. The authors suspect that the differing results between P7 and P16 rats may have something to do with the change in $GABA_A$ receptor activity. Whereas $GABA_A$ receptors in P0–P10 rats are excitatory, they change to inhibitory receptors in P16 rats. This is linked primarily to a change in developmental expression of the K^+-Cl^- cotransporter KCC2, actively removing intracellular Cl^- from neurons [16]. Exposure of P7 rats to volatile anesthetics might overly activate cells via excitatory $GABA_A$ receptors and lead to a decrease in dendrite spines as well as to neuroapoptosis.

Although several investigators have reported alarming results of anesthesia-induced neurotoxicity in the developing brain, questions remain as to whether the study designs are in fact relevant to clinical practice. Anesthetics are administered to patients to alleviate pain perception; however, the vast majority of studies have tested the effects of volatile anesthetics in the absence of painful stimuli. Shu and colleagues attempted to address this issue by testing the effects of volatile anesthetics in the presence or absence of painful stimuli [17]. They administered 70% nitrous oxide and 0.75% isoflurane to P7 rats for 6 h with or without 5% formalin injection or surgical incision to the paw. Anesthetics enhanced the degree of apoptosis. Despite the fact that anesthetics have anti-inflammatory properties, an increased level of IL-1β was found in the brain, and this was suggested as the underlying mechanism for increased apoptosis. Although it is unclear whether the increased IL-1β was a direct result of exposure to isoflurane or nitrous oxide alone or a combination of both, this is the first study to test the effects of anesthetics in the setting of painful stimulation. Studies assessing the effects of painful stimuli should be carried out for other volatile anesthetics.

Several groups have also studied intravenous anesthetics in neonatal rats. Hayashi and colleagues assessed the effects of ketamine, used as an adjunctive for premedication and for anesthesia induction and maintenance as well as postoperative pain, in P7 rats [18]. They administered either a single-dose injection (25, 50, or 75 mg/kg) or a repeated injection of 25 mg/kg for seven doses and analyzed histologic sections for neuroapoptosis [18]. They found that only the latter group (25 mg/kg ketamine for seven doses) showed significant apoptosis. The same group also injected five doses of 5, 10, or 20 mg/kg ketamine over a period of 6 h and found that repeated injection of 20 mg/kg ketamine was associated with neuronal apoptosis immediately after the last injection [19]. They also showed that aberrant cell cycle reentry was responsible for neuroapoptosis [19]. Fredriksson and colleagues studied P10 mice exposed to a single injection of ketamine (25 mg/kg) [20]. There was no increase in neuronal apoptosis and no impairment in neurocognitive function, consistent with prior studies. All of these studies were performed in the absence of painful stimuli. In this setting, repeated high-dose ketamine induced neuroapoptosis.

Anand and colleagues examined the effects of painful stimuli alone or combined with ketamine [21]. They induced painful stimulation with a single injection of 4% formalin in P1, P7, and P14 rats or by a daily injection of formalin from P1 to P4 with or without 5 mg/kg ketamine. This ketamine dose is commonly used in clinical practice. A single injection of formalin in P1 and P7 rats, as well as repeated injection, induced neuroapoptosis, which was attenuated by low-dose ketamine.

Liu and colleagues examined the effects of pain stimulation induced by a single injection of complete Freund's adjuvant (CFA), repeated high-dose ketamine injection (five 20 mg/kg doses over a period of 6 h), or both on brain apoptosis in P7 rats [22]. Ketamine induced significant apoptosis, which was attenuated by concurrent pain stimulation, even though CFA-induced painful simulation itself resulted in a small enhancement of neuronal apoptosis [22]. These results are in contrast to those with painful stimulation and isoflurane. Whether this represents differential effects of these drugs in the setting of painful stimulation needs to be clarified.

The effect of ketamine on synapse formation has also been studied. De Roo and colleagues reported that ketamine increases spine density in P16 rats [23], but there are as yet no reported studies of spine density in younger rats. Histologic analysis of apoptosis appears to be the mainstay in ketamine studies, and functional assessments have been scarce. Given that neuroapoptosis has been observed only in response to high-dose, repeated ketamine injection, the clinical relevance of ketamine-induced neurotoxicity remains to be determined.

Propofol is a commonly used intravenous drug in surgery, procedures, and sedation in the intensive care unit (ICU). In 1999, the FDA approved the use of propofol in infants as young as 3 months of age. Cattano and colleagues injected a single dose of propofol (25, 50, 100, 200, or 300 mg/kg) in P5–P7 mice and examined histologic sections at 6 h after injection [24]. Propofol at 50 mg/kg or greater induced neuroapoptosis. However, they did not evaluate functional outcomes. Karen and colleagues examined P6 rat brains after propofol injection (three 30 mg/kg doses) [25]. Histology was performed at 6, 12, and 24 h after the first injection. Propofol injection was associated with transiently increased apoptosis, peaking at 12 h, and a downregulation of neurotrophin mRNA. Propofol-treated rats showed a significant increase rather than a decrease in locomotion and travel distance at P30, and there were no changes in behavior at P120. In addition, there were no changes in memory. Fredriksson et al. tested the effects of 10 and 60 mg/kg propofol in P10 mice and observed no significant differences in behavior at P55 [20]. De Roo et al. tested the effect of propofol on synaptogenesis in P16 mice and found that propofol increased spine density via an increased rate of protrusion formation and enhanced stabilization of newly formed spines, as seen with volatile anesthetics and ketamine [23]. However, its effect on spine density on younger rats has not been reported. Propofol might induce neuroapoptosis at clinically relevant dosages, but functional data on propofol-induced neurotoxicity are rather scarce at present.

Whereas ketamine and propofol act on NMDA receptors and $GABA_A$ receptors, respectively, both of which are critical for neurogenesis, dexmedetomidine is pharmacologically different, acting as an α2-adrenergic receptor agonist. This drug is rarely used as a sole anesthetic in surgical anesthesia, but it can be used as sedation in the ICU. Sanders and colleagues examined the effect of dexmedetomidine in conjunction with isoflurane anesthesia [26]. P7 rats were exposed to 0.75% isoflurane for 6 h with or without dexmedetomidine (three doses of 1, 10, or 25 μg/kg). Dexmedetomidine dose-dependently attenuated isoflurane-induced apoptosis in the hippocampus, thalamus, and cortex. Isoflurane induced memory impairment at P40, which was also attenuated by the administration of dexmedetomidine. At these doses, dexmedetomidine itself did not induce pathologic neuroapoptosis. Li and colleagues investigated the mechanism whereby dexmedetomidine attenuates volatile anesthetic-induced neuroapoptosis [27]. They pretreated P7 rats with various concentrations of dexmedetomidine and exposed them to 0.75% isoflurane or 1.2% sevoflurane for 6 h. Isoflurane, but not sevoflurane, induced neuronal apoptosis, and dexmedetomidine pretreatment dose-dependently inhibited isoflurane-induced neuroapoptosis by preserving the activity of the phosphoinositide 3-kinase (PI3K)/Akt pathway. The PI3K/Akt pathway is critical for the cell cycle. On the basis of these studies, dexmedetomidine was suggested to attenuate neurotoxicity by reducing the requirement for other anesthetics, as well as by its direct effect in attenuating neuroapoptosis [4]. However, high-dose dexmedetomidine alone (four doses of 50 μg/kg i.p.) can induce apoptosis in P7 rats (personal communication with Dr. Sulpicio G. Soriano, Boston Children's Hospital), and the benefit of dexmedetomidine needs to be clarified.

Aside from ketamine, propofol, and dexmedetomidine, other intravenous anesthetics have not been studied much. Thiopental, once a popular induction drug and used as maintenance in some instances, is no longer produced, and etomidate is unlikely to be used as maintenance, owing to its effect of adrenal suppression.

3.3.2 Primate Studies

The studies in rodents raised significant concern regarding the administration of anesthetics to the developing brain. Although rodent studies are easier to perform and potentially provide in-depth information on gene modulation methods, studies in larger animals closer to humans are necessary.

Several groups have examined the effects of anesthetics in nonhuman primates. Dobbing and Sands suggested that the brains of rhesus monkeys at P6 are developmentally similar to the brains of human infants at 4–6 months of age [28]. Accordingly, monkeys at P5–P6 have been used in the majority of studies.

Isoflurane is the only volatile anesthetic tested thus far in nonhuman primates. Brambrink and colleagues exposed P6 rhesus macaques to 0.7–1.5% isoflurane to obtain surgical levels of anesthesia for 5 h [29]. They inspected white matter at 3 h after the end of exposure and found that the isoflurane-treated group showed significant apoptosis of neuronal cells. This group later examined gray matter in the same study design and found that oligodendrocytes in the gray matter were apoptotic as well [30]. Oligodendrocytes are critical for myelinogenesis, and this finding suggests that cells other than neurons may be involved in isoflurane-induced neurotoxicity. Zou and colleagues exposed P5–P6 rhesus monkeys to 70% nitrous oxide, 1% isoflurane, or both for 8 h [31]. The combination of nitrous oxide and isoflurane induced significant neuronal apoptosis, but either alone did not induce significant apoptosis. Whether 1% isoflurane was below the threshold for inducing apoptosis needs to be clarified. Both 1 and 1.5% isoflurane are in the clinically relevant range, and determining if there is a safe isoflurane dosage threshold is important. It is worth mentioning that no functional outcomes have been reported in any studies of isoflurane in nonhuman primates, and this needs to be addressed.

Ketamine and propofol have been tested as intravenous anesthetics in nonhuman primates. Creeley and colleagues tested the effect of 5 h of propofol exposure in P6 rhesus macaques [32]. Histology revealed increased apoptosis in response to propofol administration. Unfortunately, no dosage regimen or functional outcomes were reported in that study. Slikker and colleagues administered a 20 mg/kg bolus followed by a 20–50 mg/kg/h infusion of ketamine for a period of 24 h in P5 or P35 rhesus monkeys [33]. The measured plasma ketamine level was 10–25 μg/mL, much higher than plasma concentrations in human patients (2–3 μg/mL). Histology revealed increased apoptosis in the P5 monkey brain but not in the P35 brain. The authors also compared the effects of 3 h versus 24 h of ketamine infusion in P5 monkeys [34]. They found that ketamine infused for 3 h caused no changes in neuroapoptosis. They also examined functional consequences in P5 rhesus monkeys who received a 20 mg/kg intramuscular ketamine injection followed by a 20–50 mg/kg/h infusion for a period of 24 h [34]. At ages 7 months to 3.5 years, they assessed learning, short-term memory, motivation, and color positioning. The ketamine-treated group showed poorer performances. The total dose of ketamine in this study was 500–1220 mg/kg by simple calculation, well above doses used in clinical practice; it is important to consider this in reference to clinical practice.

Do all anesthetics increase neuroapoptosis in similar brain regions? Brambrink and colleagues noted that isoflurane induces apoptosis with a much broader distribution than does ketamine [35]. This may have to do with differences in direct effects of these drugs, but other factors may be involved. For example, Martin and colleagues examined physiologic parameters in P5–P7 rhesus macaques during isoflurane, ketamine, or propofol anesthesia [36]. Doses of 1.5–3.0% isoflurane (mean, 2.3%), a 20 mg/kg bolus followed by a 20–55 mg/kg/h infusion of ketamine (mean, 38.8 mg/kg/h), or a 2 mg/kg bolus followed by a 24–37 mg/kg/h infusion of propofol (mean, 32.5 mg/kg/h) were administered for a period of 5 h. Isoflurane anesthesia was associated with lower mean blood pressure compared to the other anesthetics. The isoflurane group received frequent boluses of crystalloid fluid to maintain mean blood pressure above 40 mm Hg. Although this isoflurane regimen differed from that in the aforementioned isoflurane-induced apoptosis study [29, 35], whether differences in hemodynamic parameters explain the distribution of neuroapoptosis may be an important issue to study in the future; this may imply the importance of maintaining perfusion pressure rather than drug type.

3.3.3 *Human Studies*

There are ample data from animal studies suggesting that anesthetics pose a risk of toxicity to the developing brain. The time frame appears to correspond to the period of peak synaptogenesis. In humans, the brain growth spurt occurs during the first 3–4 years of life. More specifically, it occurs near the time of birth in the primary sensorimotor cortex, at 9 months of age in the temporal cortex, and at 3 years of age in the prefrontal cortex [37]. Various investigators have retrospectively examined the possible association of anesthesia with learning and behavioral abnormalities. Thus far, there are no studies using any kind of imaging modality.

Wilder and colleagues performed a population-based cohort study in children born between 1976 and 1982 in Rochester, Minnesota [38]. Of the 5357 subjects, 593 received general anesthesia before the age of 4 years. The development of reading and mathematics learning disabilities was assessed. A single exposure to anesthesia was not associated with an increased risk of learning disabilities (hazard ratio [HR], 1.0). However, the HR was 1.59 for two exposures and 2.60 for three or more exposures. Flick and colleagues used the same database and examined 350 children exposed to anesthesia before the age of 2 years [39]. The analysis was adjusted for comorbidities. Multiple exposures to anesthetics significantly increased the risk of mathematics, reading, or writing learning disabilities (HR, 2.16), but a single exposure did not (HR, 1.10). An association of anesthetic exposure before the age of 2 years with the receipt of an individualized education program for speech-language impairment was observed in children with multiple exposures but not for a single exposure. This group also examined the association of anesthetic exposure before the age of 2 years with the development of attention-deficit/hyperactivity disorder (ADHD) in the same population [40]. They found that multiple exposures were associated with a risk of ADHD (HR, 1.95), but a single exposure was not (HR, 1.18). Halothane and nitrous oxide were the main drugs administered as anesthetics to that population. Halothane is no longer a mainstay anesthetic drug because it is associated with bradycardia and other arrhythmias. In addition, monitoring, such as pulse oximetry, was not available in late 1970s and early 1980s, and whether undetected desaturation during anesthesia was associated with these results is unclear.

Hansen and colleagues performed a retrospective study of Danish birth cohorts born during the period 1986–1990 [41]. They compared academic performance at ninth grade for all children who underwent inguinal hernia repair before the age of 1 year (2689 children) to a randomly selected, age-matched, 5% population sample (14,575 children). No single, relatively brief anesthetic exposure in connection with hernia repair in infancy reduced academic performance (HR, 1.18).

Bartels and colleagues examined twins born between 1986 and 1995 using the Netherlands Twin Registry [42]. They examined twins who underwent anesthesia before the age of 3 years, and educational achievement and cognitive problems were assessed via standardized tests and teacher rating near the age of 12 years. Twins who were exposed to anesthesia before age 3 had significantly lower educational achievement scores and significantly more cognitive problems than twins who were not, but the unexposed co-twins from discordant pairs did not differ from twins not exposed to anesthesia. The authors concluded, "there is no evidence for a causal relationship between anesthesia administration and later learning-related outcomes. Rather there is evidence for early anesthesia being a marker of an individual's vulnerability for later learning problems, regardless of their exposure to anesthesia." These studies did not support the idea that anesthetics induce learning disabilities.

Ing and colleagues used the database from the Western Australian Pregnancy Cohort (Raine) Study, which included 2868 children born during the period 1989–1992 [43]. Excluding 260 children lost to follow-up, 321 children were exposed to anesthesia before the age of 3 years, and 2287 were unexposed. The authors evaluated the association between exposure to anesthesia before age 3 and outcomes in language, cognitive function, motor skills, and behavior at age 10. Exposure to anesthesia was associated with an increased risk of disability in listening comprehension (HR, 1.87), speaking ability (HR, 1.72), and cognition (HR, 1.69). Increased risks were also noted in language and cognition, even after a single exposure to anesthetics (HR, 2.41 and 1.73, respectively). However, there were no differences in visual tracking and attention, fine and gross motor functions, or behavior. Unfortunately, information regarding the anesthetics used was not available.

DiMaggio and colleagues performed a retrospective cohort analysis of children born during the period 1991–2002 and enrolled in the New York State Medicaid Program [44]. A total of 383 children who underwent inguinal hernia repair during the first 3 years of life were matched with control subjects. They found that children who underwent hernia repair before age 3 were more than twice as likely as children in the control group to receive subsequent diagnosis of a developmental or behavioral disorder (HR, 2.3). That group used the same database to perform a retrospective study of a sibling birth cohort born during the period 1999–2005 [45]. A total of 304 children without a history of developmental or behavioral disorders who underwent surgery before the age of 3 years were compared to children who did not. The HR for any developmental or behavioral disorder associated with any exposure to anesthesia before age 3 was 1.1 for one operation, 2.9 for two operations, and 4.0 for more than three operations. Studies of this database suggest that anesthetic exposure may be associated with learning or developmental problems.

The studies described thus far were performed in the United States, Europe, and Australia. Ko and colleagues examined children born during the period 2001–2005 using the national health insurance research database of Taiwan and compared 3293 children with anesthesia exposure before the age of 3 years to children without to examine the association of early-life anesthesia exposure with the risk of ADHD [46]. The adjusted HR of developing ADHD for single and multiple anesthesia exposures was 1.11 and 0.96, respectively.

Although some studies suggest an association of anesthesia exposure with risk of learning and developmental disabilities, others do not support. Even if there is an association, repeated, early anesthetic exposure may be simply a marker of vulnerability for later learning disorder, particularly considering the result of the study by Barterls et al. [42]. At this point, there is no clear evidence to state unequivocally that early exposure to anesthetics worsens neurocognitive function. Therefore, until there is a clear answer, it is important to provide adequate anesthesia for patients with the use of available drugs.

3.3.4 Ongoing Clinical Studies

Prospective studies are currently being performed to determine if anesthetics affect brain development. Table 3.2 lists ongoing clinical studies. The aim of the Pediatric Anesthesia and NeuroDevelopment Assessment (PANDA) study is to perform prospective neuropsychologic assessment in anesthetic-exposed and non-exposed siblings [47]. Enrolled subjects have an ASA physical status score of 1 or 2. The exposed siblings receive anesthesia for inguinal hernia repair before the age of 3 years, and the unexposed siblings have no anesthesia before age 3. The neurodevelopmental outcome measures include global intelligence quotient (IQ) and targeted areas of neurocognitive function, such as attention, memory, behavior, and motor function, tested at the ages of 8 and 15 years. The General

Table 3.2 Ongoing clinical studies investigating the effects of anesthesia on the developing human brain

Study	Objective/comparison	Evaluation	Progress status
PANDA study [47]	Received GA before age 3 years for inguinal hernia repair/unexposed siblings	IQ, attention, memory, behavior, and motor function at ages 8 and 15 years	Pilot study completed [50]; under enrollment
GAS study [48]	Received GA before age 6 months for inguinal hernia repair/received spinal anesthesia	Developmental test at age 2 years; neurodevelopmental and intelligence tests at age 5 years	Expected completion 2015–2016
MASK study [49]	Received GA before age 3 years (1994–2007)/propensity score-matched study	Neuropsychologic test between ages 8 and 19 or 15 and 19 years	Evaluations conducted 2012–2016

GA general anesthesia, *GAS* General Anesthesia and Spinal, *IQ* intelligence quotient, *MASK* Mayo Anesthesia Safety in Kids, *PANDA* Pediatric Anesthesia and NeuroDevelopment Assessment

Anesthesia and Spinal (GAS) study is a randomized trial to compare the effects of general and spinal anesthesia on neurodevelopmental outcomes and apnea in infants younger than 6 months of age undergoing inguinal hernia repair [48]. Patients were randomly assigned to receive general anesthesia or spinal anesthesia for inguinal hernia repair, and enrollment was completed in 2013. The children undergo developmental testing at age 2 and neurodevelopmental and intelligence testing at age 5. The Mayo Anesthesia Safety in Kids (MASK) study is a population-based, propensity score-matched study to evaluate potential anesthetic effects in children born in Rochester, Minnesota, during the period 1994–2007 [49]. Existing medical records are used to identify children who were exposed to general anesthesia before age 3. Children with multiple, single, and no anesthesia exposure are sampled for neuropsychologic testing between the ages of 8 and 12 years or 15 and 19 years. Data from these studies will likely become available within the next 5 years.

3.4 Conclusion

Further data are necessary to make any kind of conclusive statement regarding the risks of anesthetic exposure in young children. Inadequate anesthesia itself is clearly a problem [51], and adequate anesthesia and analgesia during surgery and procedures are essential in daily clinical practice. How best to provide adequate anesthesia needs to be revisited continuously, but at this moment, there is no conclusive evidence to state that anesthetics themselves worsen the developing brain in humans, and we should use good judgment regarding the adequate and safe administration of anesthetics, as we do regularly. However, it is also important to identify clear indications for surgery or procedures requiring anesthesia in young children and to avoid unnecessary anesthetics in this potentially vulnerable population.

References

1. Ikonomidou C, Bosch F, Miksa M et al (1999) Blockade of NMDA receptors and apoptotic neurodegeneration in the developing brain. Science 283:70–74
2. Ikonomidou C, Bittigau P, Ishimaru MJ et al (2000) Ethanol-induced apoptotic neurodegeneration and fetal alcohol syndrome. Science 287:1056–1060
3. Jevtovic-Todorovic V, Hartman RE, Izumi Y et al (2003) Early exposure to common anesthetic agents causes widespread neurodegeneration in the developing rat brain and persistent learning deficits. J Neurosci 23:876–882
4. Rappaport BA, Suresh S, Hertz S et al (2015) Anesthetic neurotoxicity—clinical implications of animal models. N Engl J Med 372:796–797. doi:10.1056/NEJMp1414786
5. Zuo Z (2012) Are volatile anesthetics neuroprotective or neurotoxic? Med Gas Res 2:10. doi:10.1186/2045-9912-2-10
6. Contestabile A (2000) Roles of NMDA receptor activity and nitric oxide production in brain development. Brain Res Brain Res Rev 32:476–509
7. Barker JL, Behar T, Li YX et al (1998) GABAergic cells and signals in CNS development. Perspect Dev Neurobiol 5:305–322
8. Yon JH, Daniel-Johnson J, Carter LB et al (2005) Anesthesia induces neuronal cell death in the developing rat brain via the intrinsic and extrinsic apoptotic pathways. Neuroscience 135:815–827
9. Head BP, Patel HH, Niesman IR et al (2009) Inhibition of p75 neurotrophin receptor attenuates isoflurane-mediated neuronal apoptosis in the neonatal central nervous system. Anesthesiology 110:813–825. doi:10.1097/ALN.0b013e31819b602b
10. Wu X, Lu Y, Dong Y et al (2012) The inhalation anesthetic isoflurane increases levels of proinflammatory TNF-α, IL-6, and IL-1β. Neurobiol Aging 33:1364–1378. doi:10.1016/j.neurobiolaging.2010.11.002
11. Loepke AW, Istaphanous GK, McAuliffe JJ 3rd et al (2009) The effects of neonatal isoflurane exposure in mice on brain cell viability, adult behavior, learning, and memory. Anesth Analg 108:90–104. doi:10.1213/ane.0b013e31818cdb29
12. Stratmann G, May LD, Sall JW et al (2009) Effect of hypercarbia and isoflurane on brain cell death and neurocognitive dysfunction in 7-day-old rats. Anesthesiology 110:849–861. doi:10.1097/ALN.0b013e31819c7140
13. Stratmann G, Sall JW, May LD et al (2009) Isoflurane differentially affects neurogenesis and long-term neurocognitive function in 60-day-old and 7-day-old rats. Anesthesiology 110:834–848. doi:10.1097/ALN.0b013e31819c463d
14. Istaphanous GK, Howard J, Nan X et al (2011) Comparison of the neuroapoptotic properties of equipotent anesthetic concentrations of desflurane, isoflurane, or sevoflurane in neonatal mice. Anesthesiology 114:578–587. doi:10.1097/ALN.0b013e3182084a70
15. Briner A, De Roo M, Dayer A et al (2010) Volatile anesthetics rapidly increase dendritic spine density in the rat medial prefrontal cortex during synaptogenesis. Anesthesiology 112:546–556. doi:10.1097/ALN.0b013e3181cd7942
16. Ben-Ari Y (2002) Excitatory actions of gaba during development: the nature of the nurture. Nat Rev Neurosci 3:728–739
17. Shu Y, Zhou Z, Wan Y et al (2012) Nociceptive stimuli enhance anesthetic-induced neuroapoptosis in the rat developing brain. Neurobiol Dis 45:743–750. doi:10.1016/j.nbd.2011.10.021
18. Hayashi H, Dikkes P, Soriano SG (2002) Repeated administration of ketamine may lead to neuronal degeneration in the developing rat brain. Paediatr Anaesth 12:770–774
19. Soriano SG, Liu Q, Li J et al (2010) Ketamine activates cell cycle signaling and apoptosis in the neonatal rat brain. Anesthesiology 112:1155–1163. doi:10.1097/ALN.0b013e3181d3e0c2
20. Fredriksson A, Pontén E, Gordh T et al (2007) Neonatal exposure to a combination of N-methyl-D-aspartate and gamma-aminobutyric acid type A receptor anesthetic agents

potentiates apoptotic neurodegeneration and persistent behavioral deficits. Anesthesiology 107:427–436
21. Anand KJ, Garg S, Rovnaghi CR et al (2007) Ketamine reduces the cell death following inflammatory pain in newborn rat brain. Pediatr Res 62:283–290
22. Liu JR, Liu Q, Li J et al (2012) Noxious stimulation attenuates ketamine-induced neuroapoptosis in the developing rat brain. Anesthesiology 117:64–71. doi:10.1097/ALN.0b013e31825ae693
23. De Roo M, Klauser P, Briner A et al (2009) Anesthetics rapidly promote synaptogenesis during a critical period of brain development. PLoS One 4:e7043. doi:10.1371/journal.pone.0007043
24. Cattano D, Young C, Straiko MM et al (2008) Subanesthetic doses of propofol induce neuroapoptosis in the infant mouse brain. Anesth Analg 106:1712–1714. doi:10.1213/ane.0b013e318172ba0a
25. Karen T, Schlager GW, Bendix I et al (2013) Effect of propofol in the immature rat brain on short- and long-term neurodevelopmental outcome. PLoS One 8:e64480. doi:10.1371/journal.pone.0064480
26. Sanders RD, Xu J, Shu Y et al (2009) Dexmedetomidine attenuates isoflurane-induced neurocognitive impairment in neonatal rats. Anesthesiology 110:1077–1085. doi:10.1097/ALN.0b013e31819daedd
27. Li Y, Zeng M, Chen W et al (2014) Dexmedetomidine reduces isoflurane-induced neuroapoptosis partly by preserving PI3K/Akt pathway in the hippocampus of neonatal rats. PLoS One 9:e93639. doi:10.1371/journal.pone.0093639
28. Dobbing J, Sands J (1979) Comparative aspects of the brain growth spurt. Early Hum Dev 3:79–83
29. Brambrink AM, Evers AS, Avidan MS et al (2010) Isoflurane-induced neuroapoptosis in the neonatal rhesus macaque brain. Anesthesiology 112:834–841. doi:10.1097/ALN.0b013e3181d049cd
30. Brambrink AM, Back SA, Riddle A et al (2012) Isoflurane-induced apoptosis of oligodendrocytes in the neonatal primate brain. Ann Neurol 72:525–535. doi:10.1002/ana.23652
31. Zou X, Liu F, Zhang X et al (2011) Inhalation anesthetic-induced neuronal damage in the developing rhesus monkey. Neurotoxicol Teratol 33:592–597. doi:10.1016/j.ntt.2011.06.003
32. Creeley C, Dikranian K, Dissen G et al (2013) Propofol-induced apoptosis of neurones and oligodendrocytes in fetal and neonatal rhesus macaque brain. Br J Anaesth 110(Suppl 1):i29–i38. doi:10.1093/bja/aet173
33. Slikker W Jr, Zou X, Hotchkiss CE et al (2007) Ketamine-induced neuronal cell death in the perinatal rhesus monkey. Toxicol Sci 98:145–158
34. Paule MG, Li M, Allen RR et al (2011) Ketamine anesthesia during the first week of life can cause long-lasting cognitive deficits in rhesus monkeys. Neurotoxicol Teratol 33:220–230. doi:10.1016/j.ntt.2011.01.001
35. Brambrink AM, Evers AS, Avidan MS et al (2012) Ketamine-induced neuroapoptosis in the fetal and neonatal rhesus macaque brain. Anesthesiology 116:372–384. doi:10.1097/ALN.0b013e318242b2cd
36. Martin LD, Dissen GA, McPike MJ et al (2014) Effects of anesthesia with isoflurane, ketamine, or propofol on physiologic parameters in neonatal rhesus macaques (Macaca mulatta). J Am Assoc Lab Anim Sci 53:290–300
37. Huttenlocher PR, Dabholkar AS (1997) Regional differences in synaptogenesis in human cerebral cortex. J Comp Neurol 387:167–178
38. Wilder RT, Flick RP, Sprung J et al (2009) Early exposure to anesthesia and learning disabilities in a population-based birth cohort. Anesthesiology 110:796–804. doi:10.1097/01.anes.0000344728.34332.5d
39. Flick RP, Katusic SK, Colligan RC et al (2011) Cognitive and behavioral outcomes after early exposure to anesthesia and surgery. Pediatrics 128:e1053–e1061. doi:10.1542/peds.2011-0351

40. Sprung J, Flick RP, Katusic SK et al (2012) Attention-deficit/hyperactivity disorder after early exposure to procedures requiring general anesthesia. Mayo Clin Proc 87:120–129. doi:10.1016/j.mayocp.2011.11.008
41. Hansen TG, Pedersen JK, Henneberg SW et al (2011) Academic performance in adolescence after inguinal hernia repair in infancy: a nationwide cohort study. Anesthesiology 114:1076–1085. doi:10.1097/ALN.0b013e31820e77a0
42. Bartels M, Althoff RR, Boomsma DI (2009) Anesthesia and cognitive performance in children: no evidence for a causal relationship. Twin Res Hum Genet 12:246–253. doi:10.1375/twin.12.3.246
43. Ing C, DiMaggio C, Whitehouse A et al (2012) Long-term differences in language and cognitive function after childhood exposure to anesthesia. Pediatrics 130:e476–e485. doi:10.1542/peds.2011-3822
44. DiMaggio C, Sun LS, Kakavouli A et al (2009) A retrospective cohort study of the association of anesthesia and hernia repair surgery with behavioral and developmental disorders in young children. J Neurosurg Anesthesiol 21:286–291. doi:10.1097/ANA.0b013e3181a71f11
45. DiMaggio C, Sun LS, Li G (2011) Early childhood exposure to anesthesia and risk of developmental and behavioral disorders in a sibling birth cohort. Anesth Analg 113:1143–1151. doi:10.1213/ANE.0b013e3182147f42
46. Ko WR, Liaw YP, Huang JY et al (2014) Exposure to general anesthesia in early life and the risk of attention deficit/hyperactivity disorder development: a nationwide, retrospective matched-cohort study. Paediatr Anaesth 24:741–748. doi:10.1111/pan.12371
47. Sun LS, Li G, Dimaggio C et al (2008) Anesthesia and neurodevelopment in children: time for an answer? Anesthesiology 109:757–761. doi:10.1097/ALN.0b013e31818a37fd
48. Davidson AJ, McCann ME, Morton NS et al (2008) Anesthesia and outcome after neonatal surgery: the role for randomized trials. Anesthesiology 109:941–944. doi:10.1097/ALN.0b013e31818e3f79
49. Gleich SJ, Flick R, Hu D et al (2015) Neurodevelopment of children exposed to anesthesia: design of the Mayo Anesthesia Safety in Kids (MASK) study. Contemp Clin Trials 41:45–54. doi:10.1016/j.cct.2014.12.020
50. Sun LS, Li G, DiMaggio CJ et al (2012) Feasibility and pilot study of the Pediatric Anesthesia NeuroDevelopment Assessment (PANDA) project. J Neurosurg Anesthesiol 24:382–388. doi:10.1097/ANA.0b013e31826a0371
51. Taddio A, Katz J, Ilersich AL et al (1997) Effect of neonatal circumcision on pain response during subsequent routine vaccination. Lancet 349:599–603

Part II
Postoperative Delirium and Cognitive Dysfunction

Chapter 4
Present Clinical Status of Postoperative Delirium (POD)

Moritoki Egi

Abstract Postoperative delirium (POD), which is considered to be a form of acute brain failure resulting from anesthesia and/or surgical operation, is one of the most common complications in postoperative patients. The clinical status of POD has been characterized as showing "fluctuating symptoms" and "deficit of attention." POD can be involved in "disorganization of behavior," "arousal changes," and "disturbance of the sleep-wake cycle." There are three types of POD: hyperactive delirium; hypoactive delirium, which has typically been unrecognized; and a mixed form, which presents with a range of both hyperactive and hypoactive symptoms.

Keywords Hypoactive • Hyperactive • Delirium • Inattention • Arousal changes

4.1 The Presence of Delirium in Postoperative Patients

Postoperative delirium (POD) is one of the most common complications in postoperative patients. Its prevalence has been reported to vary from 5% [1] to 50% [2], according to the study case-mix and type of operation. Delirium is more likely to occur in elderly patients [2]. As the number of operations in elderly patients is likely to increase, and as radical operations, which have a higher risk of delirium, are now being indicated for elderly patients, the issue of delirium is becoming more problematic in perioperative medicine. In this regard, it is relevant for clinicians to be alert to the presence of delirium so that they can provide optimally for its prevention and treatment.

Delirium is characterized by the acute onset of changed mental status, with inattention, disorganized thinking, or an altered level of consciousness; the symptoms show a fluctuating course [3], and the condition is common in critically ill patients [4]. POD is defined as delirium that occurs postoperatively. POD is considered to be

---

M. Egi, M.D.
Department of Anesthesiology, Kobe University Hospital,
7-5-2 Kusunoki-cho, Chuo-ku, Kobe, Hyogo 650-0017, Japan
e-mail: moriori@tg8.so-net.ne.jp

Y. Morimoto (ed.), *Anesthesia and Neurotoxicity*,
DOI 10.1007/978-4-431-55624-4_4

a form of acute brain failure (a postoperative organ failure), resulting from either anesthesia, an operation, or both. Although surgical operations, anesthetics, and analgesics can contribute to POD, the condition is not associated only with emergence from anesthesia; it often occurs between postoperative days 1 and 3. Although patients with POD commonly recover within a short period [5], patients with POD, compared with patients without this condition, are more likely to die or to develop dementia, and require institutionalization [6].

The first relevant step to prevent and treat POD is to recognize its presence. Therefore, clinicians should be aware of the clinical status of POD.

4.2 The Difference Between Dementia and Delirium

Dementia and delirium may seem to be difficult to distinguish. Indeed, some patients have both dementia and delirium. It is also true that the presence of dementia is a risk factor for delirium. However, to understand what delirium is, comparisons between delirium and dementia are useful. Table 4.1 shows comparisons of the features of dementia and delirium. Patients with dementia may have a progressive decline of memory and other cognitive skills, whereas the onset of delirium occurs acutely (within a short time). Dementia usually occurs chronically, and gradually worsens over time. Patients with dementia show impaired memory in the early stage. Patients with delirium have impaired ability to stay focused or maintain attention. The symptoms of delirium may fluctuate within a day, whereas symptoms of dementia are usually constant over a day.

4.3 Risk of and Precipitating Factors for POD

There are a number of risk factors for POD, with five major factors: age more than 65 years, dementia, poor vision, poor hearing, and infection. It is also known that physiological stressors that are determined mainly by the extent of the operation are risk factors for POD as well [7]. Table 4.2 shows a list of risk factors reported in the best practice statement from the American Geriatrics Society. The greater the number of risk factors, the higher is the risk of POD. It is also reported that POD is more likely to occur after emergency surgery rather than after elective surgery.

Table 4.1 Comparison of dementia and delirium

	Dementia	Delirium
Onset	Chronic	Acute
Impairment	Memory	Attention
Fluctuation of symptoms	Symptoms constant over a daily period	Symptoms fluctuate frequently within 1 day
Prognosis	Chronically worsens	Possible recovery

Table 4.2 Known risk factors for postoperative dementia (POD)

Age greater than 65 years
Cognitive impairment
Severe illness or comorbidity burden
Hearing or vision impairment
Current hip fracture
Presence of infection
Inadequately controlled pain
Depression
Alcohol use
Sleep deprivation or disturbance
Renal insufficiency
Anemia
Hypoxia or hypercarbia
Poor nutrition
Dehydration
Electrolyte abnormalities (hyper- or hyponatremia)
Poor functional status
Immobilization or limited mobility
Polypharmacy and use of psychotropic medications
(benzodiazepines, anticholinergics, antihistamines, antipsychotics)
Risk of urinary retention or constipation
Presence of urinary catheter
Aortic procedures

Reference [7]

POD is commonly the consequence of physiological stressors such as the surgery, and predisposing factors [2]. Postoperative precipitating factors for POD may include environmental factors, infection, metabolic derangement, and substance withdrawal [2, 7, 8] (Table 4.3).

4.4 Pathophysiology of POD

Although a number of risk factors for POD have been reported, the pathophysiology of the condition is poorly understood. Several hypotheses have been put forward to explain this condition. The anesthesia and the operation may affect neurotransmitter levels and cause mental dysfunction. Acetylcholine is a crucial neurotransmitter that may play a relevant role in awareness and arousal. It is well known that older patients are deficient in acetylcholine; therefore, they would be relatively more sensitive to anticholinergic drugs. Table 4.4 provides a list of possible neurotransmitters that may contribute to the occurrence of POD [9]; their features include cholinergic inhibition, serotonin deficiency, dopamine activation [10], gamma-aminobutyric acid (GABA) activity [11], and melatonin activity [12]; the involvement of these features in POD is not fully understood [9].

Table 4.3 Precipitating factors for POD

Environmental factors
Inadequately controlled pain
Sleep disturbance
Use of physical restraints
Infection
Delirium-inducing medications
Drugs with anticholinergic properties
Corticosteroids
Meperidine
Sedative hypnotics
Metabolic derangement
Hypoxia
Acidosis
Electrolyte derangement
Hypoglycemia
Dehydration
Acute blood loss anemia
Hypotension/shock
Substance withdrawal
Alcohol
Benzodiazepines
Illicit drugs

Reference [7]

Table 4.4 Neurotransmitters that may contribute to POD

Acetylcholine
GABA
Glutamate
Dopamine
Serotonin
Cortisol

Reference [9]

4.5 Clinical Characteristics of POD

POD is considered to be a form of acute brain failure resulting from anesthesia and/or operation. The clinical status of POD has been characterized as showing "fluctuating symptoms" and "deficit of attention." POD can be involved in "disorganization of behavior," "arousal changes," and "disturbance of the sleep-wake cycle." Table 4.5 lists the general symptoms of POD reported in the best practice statement from the American Geriatrics Society [7].

Table 4.5 General symptoms associated with POD

• Changes in level of arousal: drowsiness, or decreased arousal, or increased arousal with hypervigilance
• Delayed awakening from anesthesia
• Abrupt change in cognitive function, including problems with attention, difficulty concentrating, new memory problems, new disorientation
• Difficulty tracking conversations and following instructions
• Thinking and speech that is disorganized, difficult to follow, slow, or rapid
• Rapidly changing emotions, easy irritability, tearfulness, uncharacteristic refusals to engage with postoperative care
• Expression of new paranoid thoughts or delusions
• New perceptual disturbances
• Motor changes, such as slowed or decreased movements, purposeless fidgeting or restlessness; new difficulties in maintaining posture, such as sitting or standing
• Sleep/wake cycle changes such as sleeping during the day and/or being awake and active at night
• Decreased appetite
• New incontinence of urine or stool
• Fluctuating symptoms and/or level of arousal over the course of minutes to hours

Reference [7]

4.5.1 Characteristics of Delirium Described in the Diagnostic and Statistical Manual Fifth Edition (DSM-5)

The DSM-5 gives us a description of the characteristics of delirium, with criteria for delirium, characterized as: (A) a disturbance in attention and awareness, (B) a disturbance that develops over a short period of time and tends to fluctuate in severity, with (C) an additional disturbance in cognition, which may not be explained by a pre-existing, established, or evolving neurocognitive disorder (Table 4.6).

4.5.2 Three Types of Postoperative Delirium

The characteristics of delirium are acute changes in mental status such as: (1) inattention, (2) disorganized thinking, and (3) an altered level of consciousness [7]. It is well known that there are three types of POD (Table 4.7). The first is hyperactive delirium; the second, which was typically unrecognized as delirium, is hypoactive delirium; and the third is mixed delirium, which presents with a range of both hyperactive and hypoactive symptoms.

Table 4.6 DSM-5[a] criteria for delirium

A. A disturbance in attention (i.e., reduced ability to direct, focus, sustain, and shift attention) and awareness (reduced orientation to the environment).
B. The disturbance develops over a short period of time (usually hours to a few days), represents a change from baseline attention and awareness, and tends to fluctuate in severity during the course of a day.
C. An additional disturbance in cognition (e.g., memory deficit; disorientation; disturbance in language, visuospatial ability, or perception).
D. The disturbances in criteria A and C are not better explained by a pre-existing, established, or evolving neurocognitive disorder and do not occur in the context of a severely reduced level of arousal, such as coma.
E. There is evidence from the history, physical examination, or laboratory findings that the disturbance is a direct physiological consequence of another medical condition, substance intoxication or withdrawal, or exposure to a toxin, or is due to multiple etiologies.

[a]American Psychiatric Association: Diagnostic and Statistical Manual of Mental Disorders. 5th edition

Table 4.7 The three types of POD

Hyperactive	"Recognized delirium"; heightened arousal, restless, agitated, and aggressive.
Hypoactive	"Rarely recognized delirium"; inactivity, decreased motor activity, and drowsiness.
Mixed	Presents with a range of both hyperactive and hypoactive symptoms.

4.5.3 Hyperactive Delirium

Hyperactive delirium, which is a "recognized delirium," presents as an agitated state. In the Richmond Agitation-Sedation Scale [13] (Table 4.8), an agitated state, i.e., frequent non-purposeful movement, is scaled as (+2); patient pulls on or removes tube(s) or catheter(s) or has aggressive behavior toward staff is scaled as (3+); and patient overtly combative or violent—immediate danger to staff—is scaled as (4+) [13]. Most medical staff are aware of hyperactive delirium and attempt to treat it. In this regard, some may believe that hyperactive delirium is equivalent to delirium or that it represents the major form of delirium.. However, hyperactive delirium is not the major form of delirium; the major form of delirium is the hypoactive form, which is described in the next section.

4.5.4 Hypoactive Delirium

Hypoactive delirium has typically been unrecognized. More than half of the patients with POD are reported to have the hypoactive form, evidenced by decreasing activity and being withdrawn. Patients with hypoactive delirium are generally calm, and lose interest in the outside world. To identify and diagnose hypoactive delirium, the

Table 4.8 The Richmond Agitation-Sedation Scale

Score	Term	Description
+4	Combative	Overtly combative or violent; immediate danger to staff
+3	Very agitated	Pulls on or removes tube(s) or catheter(s) or has aggressive behavior toward staff
+2	Agitated	Frequent non-purposeful movement, or patient-ventilator dyssynchrony
+1	Restless	Anxious or apprehensive but movements not aggressive or vigorous
0	Alert and calm	
−1	Drowsy	Not fully alert, but has sustained (more than 10 s) awakening with eye contact, in response to voice
−2	Light sedation	Briefly (less than 10 s) awakens with eye contact in response to voice
−3	Moderate sedation	Any movement (but no eye contact) in response to voice
−4	Deep sedation	No response to voice, but any movement in response to physical stimulation
−5	Unarousable	No response to voice or physical stimulation

Reference [13]

confusion assessment method for the ICU (CAM-ICU) or the intensive care delirium screening checklist (ICDSC) [14] has been used.

4.5.5 Disruption of the Sleep-Wake Cycle

Disturbance of the sleep-wake cycle is frequently observed in patients with delirium; these disturbances involve insomnia, somnolence, sleep fragmentation, or sleep-wake cycle reversal, which may reflect alterations of circadian rhythm. The relationship of circadian disturbances to the characteristic fluctuating severity of delirium symptoms over a 24-h period or to motor disturbance is unknown.

4.6 Clinical Consequences of POD

Patients with POD are more likely to have known risk factors and to be critically ill. Therefore, it is reasonable to conclude that patients with POD will have poor consequences compared with those without POD. Although patients with POD commonly recover within a short period [5], these patients are more likely to die or develop dementia and require institutionalization [6].

POD has also been reported to be associated with a significant decline in cognitive ability during the first year after cardiac surgery, with a trajectory characterized by an initial decline and prolonged impairment [15].

References

1. Dasgupta M, Dumbrell AC (2006) Preoperative risk assessment for delirium after noncardiac surgery: a systematic review. J Am Geriatr Soc 54:1578–1589
2. Inouye SK, Westendorp RG, Saczynski JS (2014) Delirium in elderly people. Lancet 383:911–922
3. Gleason OC (2003) Delirium. Am Fam Physician 67:1027–1034
4. Deiner S, Silverstein JH (2009) Postoperative delirium and cognitive dysfunction. Br J Anaesth 103(Suppl. 1):i41–i46
5. Brauer C, Morrison RS, Silberzweig SB, Siu AL (2000) The cause of delirium in patients with hip fracture. Arch Intern Med 160:1856–1860
6. Bickel H, Gradinger R, Kochs E, Forstl H (2008) High risk of cognitive and functional decline after postoperative delirium. A three-year prospective study. Dement Geriatr Cogn Disord 26:26–31
7. American Geriatrics Society Expert Panel on Postoperative Delirium in Older Adults (2014) Postoperative delirium in older adults: best practice statement from the American Geriatrics Society. J Am Coll Surg 220:136–48.e1
8. Robinson TN, Eiseman B (2008) Postoperative delirium in the elderly: diagnosis and management. Clin Interv Aging 3:351–355
9. Flacker JM, Lipsitz LA (1999) Neural mechanisms of delirium: current hypotheses and evolving concepts. J Gerontol A Biol Sci Med Sci 54:B239–B246
10. Marcantonio ER, Rudolph JL, Culley D, Crosby G, Alsop D, Inouye SK (2006) Serum biomarkers for delirium. J Gerontol A Biol Sci Med Sci 61:1281–1286
11. Yoshitaka S, Egi M, Kanazawa T, Toda Y, Morita K (2014) The association of plasma gamma-aminobutyric acid concentration with postoperative delirium in critically ill patients. Crit Care Resusc 16:269–273
12. Yoshitaka S, Egi M, Morimatsu H, Kanazawa T, Toda Y, Morita K (2013) Perioperative plasma melatonin concentration in postoperative critically ill patients: its association with delirium. J Crit Care 28:236–242
13. Ely EW, Truman B, Shintani A, Thomason JW, Wheeler AP, Gordon S, Francis J, Speroff T, Gautam S, Margolin R, Sessler CN, Dittus RS, Bernard GR (2003) Monitoring sedation status over time in ICU patients: reliability and validity of the Richmond Agitation-Sedation Scale (RASS). JAMA 289:2983–2991
14. Gusmao-Flores D, Salluh JI, Chalhub RA, Quarantini LC (2012) The confusion assessment method for the intensive care unit (CAM-ICU) and intensive care delirium screening checklist (ICDSC) for the diagnosis of delirium: a systematic review and meta-analysis of clinical studies. Crit Care 16:R115
15. Saczynski JS, Marcantonio ER, Quach L, Fong TG, Gross A, Inouye SK, Jones RN (2012) Cognitive trajectories after postoperative delirium. N Engl J Med 367:30–39

Chapter 5
Present Clinical Status of Postoperative Cognitive Dysfunction in Cardiovascular Surgery

Kazuyoshi Ishida, Atsuo Yamashita, Satoshi Yamashita, and Mishiya Matsumoto

Abstract Postoperative cognitive dysfunction (POCD) is one of the serious cerebral complications that occur after cardiac and major vascular surgery, leading to low quality of life and poor prognosis of the patients. POCD has been comprehensively investigated in coronary artery bypass grafting surgery with cardiopulmonary bypass (CPB) to elucidate its risk factors and to seek a better management that can reduce the development of POCD. However, in patients with coronary artery disease, the long-term (>6 months) incidence rate of cognitive dysfunction did not differ significantly in four treatment groups (coronary artery bypass grafting surgery with, or without CPB, percutaneous coronary intervention, and drug therapy plus follow-up observation). These findings suggest that surgery and CPB affect cognitive impairment for only about 6 months after surgery. On the other hand, there is no well-designed study for POCD with sufficient number of patients in valvular and major vascular surgery. Future challenges need the elucidation of long-term incidence rate of POCD in these surgeries and should include the patients with less invasive procedure such as transcatheter aortic valve implantation and thoracic endovascular aortic repair surgery.

Keywords Postoperative cognitive dysfunction • Coronary artery bypass grafting surgery • Cardiopulmonary bypass • Valvular surgery • Major vascular surgery

5.1 Introduction

Postoperative cognitive dysfunction (POCD) is one of the serious cerebral complications leading to low quality of life in patients after surgery. POCD is also known to affect patient prognosis, and various factors are involved in its onset.

K. Ishida (✉) • A. Yamashita • S. Yamashita • M. Matsumoto
Department of Anesthesiology, Yamaguchi University Graduate School of Medicine, 1-1-1 Minamikogushi, Ube, Yamaguchi 755-8505, Japan
e-mail: ishid002@yamaguchi-u.ac.jp

Y. Morimoto (ed.), *Anesthesia and Neurotoxicity*,
DOI 10.1007/978-4-431-55624-4_5

Cardiopulmonary bypass (CPB) is regarded as the major cause of POCD because of its adverse effect on cerebral function by scattering intracardiac air and emboli due to aortic cannulation and aortic cross-clamping. In addition, CPB procedure may produce cerebral hypoperfusion, anemia, blood brain barrier impairment, and severe systemic inflammation that could induce brain inflammation. Therefore, since the 1990s, many studies have been done for the evaluation of the risk factors and/or better management of CPB to reduce the development of POCD in the patients who underwent on-pump coronary artery bypass grafting surgery (ONCAB). According to a review published in 2000, the incidence rate of POCD in ONCAB was reported from 30 to 79% [1].

Recent studies have investigated the incidence rate of cognitive dysfunction and have compared the results between ONCAB and coronary artery bypass graft surgical without CPB (OPCAB), percutaneous coronary intervention (PCI), or drug therapy plus follow-up observation (FCA) in patients with coronary artery disease. However, the long-term (>6 months) incidence rate of cognitive dysfunction did not differ significantly in four treatment groups, suggesting that surgery and CPB affect cognitive impairment for only about 6 months after surgery.

In Japan, while the number of surgeries for coronary artery disease has been decreasing because of advances in PCI based technology, the number of valvular and major vascular surgeries is rising [2]. Compared with ONCAB, the production and scattering of emboli to the brain occur more frequently in valvular and major vascular surgeries. In addition, selective cerebral perfusion is necessary during CPB in major vascular surgery, leading to insufficient blood flow to the brain. Therefore, the evaluation of development of POCD in valvular and major vascular surgery may become more important.

In this chapter, we review the incidence rate and risk factors of POCD in ONCAB and describe the trials for reducing its occurrence. In addition, we also indicate the comparison study that shows the differences in development of cognitive dysfunction after ONCAB, OPCAB, PCI, and FCA patients. Furthermore, we review the incidence rate of POCD in valvular and major vascular surgeries. We have listed as many references as possible in tables for easier access to the representative articles used in this chapter.

5.2 Evaluation of POCD

Because POCD is not treated as a disease, it is not included in the Diagnostic and Statistical Manual of Mental Disorders (DSM)-5 published by the American Psychiatric Association, meaning that there is no appropriate diagnostic criteria for it. Therefore, POCD is evaluated based on scores from some neuropsychological test (NT)s in ombination. Although consensus has been reached on which NTs should be used [3], only half of the studies evaluating the POCD have used these agreed-upon NTs [4]. In addition, these studies used various methods to analyze changes in the NT scores, and various time points of evaluation, making inter-study comparison of POCD incidence rate extremely difficult. In general, POCD is considered to be present when ≥2 NTs or cognitive domains indicate impairment of cognition event at ≥1 week after surgery. The evaluation of POCD is difficult when NTs are performed within a week of surgery because of the postoperative pain, residual effects of anesthesia, and postoperative delirium. Usually, POCD occurring within 3 months of surgery is defined as early POCD. Impairment of NT score is judged based on ≥1 standard deviation (SD) change or ≥20% change of preoperative NT scores (because 1 SD is often equal to 20% change in the scores in NTs), or a change of ≥1.96 points in *Z*-scores compared with the control group or using the reliable change index. However, there are some studies that assessed POCD only by comparing the pre- and post-operative mean NT scores or by showing the numbers of NTs that was worsened postoperatively.

Table 5.1 shows representative articles investigating the incidence rate of POCD in ONCAB [5–27]. Due to the use of different NTs and different time points of evaluation in these studies, the incidence rate of POCD ranged greatly from 0 to 81%, including two studies reporting no development of POCD [5, 6]. Raymond et al. [7] showed that the incidence rate of POCD on postoperative day 5 differed (3.6, 4.2, or 7.7%) when different evaluations were performed (reduction in scores ≥1 SD or 20%, or evaluating with reliable change index, respectively). In addition, according to the statistical concept of regression toward the mean that promotes scores from the second test to be converged with the initial mean scores, the NT scores of patients with ONCAB revealed decrease in those with higher preoperative scores but increase in those with lower preoperative scores at 3 months after surgery [8]. This suggests that caution must be paid when evaluating POCD performed only based on decreasing NT scores in patients who had high preoperative scores.

Only a few studies have investigated which domains in NT are vulnerable. By focusing on this issue, Kneebone et al. [9] showed that memory domain of spared and retrieval were affected (48% and 35% of patients, respectively) more than memory domain of encoding and storage (17%).

5.3 Development of POCD in ONCAB

5.3.1 Risk Factors

Many studies have investigated the risk factors for POCD (Table 5.1, middle rows) [10–24]. The risk factors involved in the development of POCD in ONCAB extracted patient background factors such as age [12, 13, 15, 18, 19], low preoperative NT scores or preexisting cognitive dysfunction [12, 14], depressive state [14], a short period of education [13, 15], and female sex [13]. Other risk factors include hypertension [13], renal dysfunction, diabetes [19], and a complicating atherosclerotic lesion of major artery [12].

Table 5.1 POCD in ONCAB

	Author Year	Number of tests	Definition of POCD	Number of cases	Timing of evaluation	Development of POCD (%)	*P*-value	Comment
Evaluation								
	Mullges [5]	8	≥1 SD, ≥2-test	52	9 days	–	–	No POCD was observed
	2002				32–65 months	0	–	
	Dupuis [6]	7	Changes in scores	332	5 months	0	–	No POCD was observed
	2006				1 year	0	–	
	Raymond [7]	9	≥1 SD · ≥20%	55/C 40	5 days	3.6 · 4.2	–	Different evaluation showed a different incidence rate of POCD
	2006		Reliable change index			7.7	–	
	Browne [8]	10	≥0.5 SD, 1 SD, and 20%	120	Discharge	–	–	The concept of the regression towards the mean was involved in the change in NT score
	1999				3 months	–	–	
	Kneebone [9]	6	*Z*-score	85/C 50	6 months	48 (spared), 35 (retrieval),	–	Different impairment rates were observed for different domain of memory functions
	2005					17 (encoding and storage)	–	
Risk factor								
	Walzer [10]	6	Changes in scores	70	2–3 days	14	–	Risk factors were defibrillation after CPB, low cardiac output, low stroke volume, and low preoperative test scores
	1997				5–9 days	–	–	
	Toner [11]		≥1 SD, 2 tests	62	1 week	48	–	Decreases in EEG power of δ, θ, α, and β waves were prominent in POCD patients
	1998				2 months	34	–	

Robson [12]	11	≥0.5 SD	102	2 months	24	–	Risk factors were age and atherosclerosis
2000		≥1 SD		,	7	–	Decrease in SjO2 was not the risk factor
Di Carlo [13]	9	Daily life activities	110(+ intracardiac)	6 months	9.1 (severe)	–	Risk factors were female sex, low education, β-blocker intake, hypertension, and low PaO2 on arrival at the ICU
2001					22 (mild-moderate)	–	
Millar [14]	1	Compared with standard value	81 (13/68)	6 days	46/12	<0.001	Risk factors were pre-existing cognitive impairment and postoperative depression
2001			(impaired/ unimpaired)	6 months	39/2	<0.001	
Newman [15]	5	≥1 SD	172	Discharge · 6 weeks	53 · 36	–	Risk factors were age, education level, and POCD at discharge
2001				6 months · 5 years	24 · 42	–	
Stygall [16]	11	*Z*-score	107	6 days	–	–	Risk factors were microembolic count and NT decline at 6 days
2003				8 weeks · 5 years	–	–	
Kruis [17]		Meta-analysis	15 references		–	–	Good association between microemboli and POCD was observed only in 5 references
2010							
Zimpfer [18]	3	≥1 SD	88/C 80	1 week	51	–	Risk factors were age, NT score decline at 4 months, and AF
2004				4 months · 3 years	49 · 50		P300 latencies in POCD patients were prolonged until 3 years postoperatively
Kadoi [19]	6	?	88	6 months	27	–	Risk factors were age, renal dysfunction, DM, and insulin dependence
2006							Decrease in SjO2 was not the risk factor
Ramlawi [20, 21]	8	≥1 SD, 25% tests	40–42 (+valvular surgery)	4–5 days	40–40.5	–	Risk factors were high values of CRP, IL-1β, IL-10, NSE, tau protein and C3a
2006							

(continued)

Table 5.1 (continued)

	Author Year	Number of tests	Definition of POCD	Number of cases	Timing of evaluation	Development of POCD (%)	*P*-value	Comment
Genetic factor								
	Tardiff [22]	7	≥20%, 20% tests	17/48	6 weeks	47	0.03–0.04	APOEε4 was associated with POCD
	1997					Whole group		
	Askar [23]	10	≥1 SD, 2 tests	17/61	Discharge	58.8/48.2	0.443	APOEε4 was not associated with POCD
	2005				3 months	29.4/37.5	0.542	
	Tagarakis [24]	3		137	1 month	95	–	No association of SOAT1 gene was observed
	2007							
Anesthetics								
	Silbert [25]	7	≥20% (1 SD), 2 tests	158/168	1 week or discharge	63/64 (14/24)	0.93 (0.031)	More patients developed POD in the low dose fentanyl (10 μg/kg) group than in the high dose (50 μg/kg) group
	2006				3 months	27/19 (13/12)	0.09 (0.24)	
	Hudetz [26]	10	≥1.96 (*Z*-score)	26/26/C 26	1 week	81/27	<0.001	Bolus dose of ketamine (0.5 mg/kg) could reduce the development of POCD
	2009							
	Schoen [27]	4	Changes in scores	60/57	6 days	–	≦0.001	Sevoflurane-based anesthesia was associated with better cognitive function than propofol
	2011			Cardiac surgery				

POCD postoperative cognitive dysfunction, *ONCAB* on-pump coronary artery bypass grafting surgery, *SD* standard deviation, *NT* neuropsychological test, *C* control, *CPB* cardiopulmonary bypass, *EEG* electroencephalogram, *SjO2* jugular bulb venous oxygen saturation, *ICU* intensive care unit, *AF* atrial fibrillation, *DM* diabetes mellitus, *CRP* C-reactive protein, *IL* interleukin, *NSE* neuron-specific enolase, *C3a* complement 3a, *APOEε4* apolipoprotein ε4, *SOAT1* sterol O-acyltransferase 1

As for intraoperative factors, the risk factors reported were ventricular fibrillation after weaning from CPB, reduced cardiac function [10], and postoperative atrial fibrillation [18]. The association between POCD and an intraoperative reduction in the jugular bulb venous oxygen saturation (SjO_2) was not clear [12, 19]. Despite a report of the association between POCD and number of intraoperative microemboli [16], this association was not supported in a review that contains 15 articles [17]. On the other hand, perioperative systemic inflammatory response [20] is currently under investigation as the primary cause of POCD in basic research studies because it could induce brain inflammation at the same time [28].

In addition, some studies showed that cognitive impairment had existed for 3–5 years in patients who had developed POCD at hospital discharge or at 4 months after ONCAB [15, 18].

The polymorphism of the apolipoprotein E (ApoE) and sterol O-acyltransferase 1 (SOAT1) genes has also been investigated for risk factors for development of POCD [22–24]. In individuals with ApoE genotype ε4, which accounts for 15% of all adult population, the removal of amyloid β-protein (Aβ) that is a causal factor of Alzheimer's disease was impaired, resulting in Aβ accumulation. Previous report showed the association between ApoE ε4 and POCD [22]. However, a recent report indicates no association between them [23]. SOAT1 is an enzyme that esterifies cholesterols in endoplasmic reticula and is involved in the production of Aβ through cholesterol esters, as in the study reporting the association between SOAT1 cytosine (C)/C type and Alzheimer's disease [29]. However, it is currently unclear whether SOAT1 is involved in POCD [24].

5.3.2 Anesthetics

Only a very few studies have investigated the association between anesthetics and POCD (Table 5.1, bottom rows) [25–27]. The $GABA_A$ agonist benzodiazepine is believed to induce postoperative delirium by impairing the production of acetylcholine in the hippocampus and basal forebrain. The inhibited production of acetylcholine may induce POCD through memory impairment. In patients who have undergone noncardiac surgery, there have been conflicting results: one study reported the involvement of a previous history of benzodiazepine administration in the development of POCD [30], whereas another study reported no association between administration of this drug as premedication and development of POCD [31]. Because benzodiazepine is used frequently in cardiovascular surgery, the association between the intraoperative use of this drug and POCD should be investigated further.

As for inhalation and intravenous anesthetics, NT scores up to 6 days after surgery were higher in patients who were administered sevoflurane-based anesthetics than in those who were administered propofol [27]. The incidence rate of POCD was slightly higher in patients undergoing ONCAB with low-dose (10 μg/kg) fentanyl than in those undergoing it with medium-dose (50 μg/kg) fentanyl [25]. The incidence rate of POCD was strongly suppressed at 1 week after a single administration of 0.5 mg/kg ketamine [26]. The same research group also reported that ketamine suppresses postoperative delirium [32], making it an attractive agent. It is thought that ketamine suppresses the incidence rate of POCD through its anti-inflammatory action.

5.3.3 Development of POCD and CPB Management

Many studies have investigated the differential effects of CPB management on POCD in ONCAB [33–50] (Table 5.2).

There are several reports on the association between POCD and body temperature management during CPB [33–39]. Normothermic CPB has been investigated intensely since the early 1990s, when a study showed the superiority of normothermic CPB (around normal body temperature) over conventional hypothermic (around 28 °C) CPB in maintaining better cardiac function. At the same time, studies were investigating cerebral infarction because of a concern about a possible increase in the incidence rate, which was followed by the research into the association between normothermic CPB and POCD. It was subsequently concluded that the incidence rate of POCD does not differ significantly whether the body temperature is maintained at 35–36 or 28 °C during CPB [34, 35]. This is thought to be because the procedures with a high risk of developing and scattering emboli to the brain, such as aortic cannulation, aortic cross-clamping, and declamping, are all performed when the body temperature is close to the normothermia. In addition, in patients undergoing hypothermic CPB, the brain is re-warmed excessively during weaning from CPB potentially cancelling out the protective effect of hypothermia. However, postoperative NT scores were worse in patients who took 37 °C normothermic CPB than those who took 28 or 32 °C CPB [33], presumably because of warming steps during CPB to keep the body temperature at 37 °C, suggesting that warming up to 37 °C may affect and impair some cognitive function in patients who undergo ONCAB. Taking this into consideration, some studies were performed maintaining the body temperature around 34 °C during and after CPB, with no active re-warming to 37 °C [36–39], and reported a reduction in development of POCD in two studies [36, 37].

As for acid-base management during CPB, an incidence rate of POCD was lower with the α-stat strategy than with the pH-stat strategy [41, 42], presumably because with α-stat, cerebral blood flow autoregulation is maintained, and

Table 5.2 POCD and CPB management in ONCAB

Author / Year	Number of tests	CPB management	Definition of POCD	Number of cases	Timing of evaluation	Development of POCD (%)	*P*-value	Comment
Temperature management								
Regragui [33]	7	28 °C vs. 32 °C vs. 37 °C	Numbers of NTs in which score was decreased	31/36/29	6 weeks	–	0.021	Disadvantage was observed in 37 °C CPB
1996								
Mora [34]	5	≤ 28 °C vs. ≥35 °C	Comparing the scores in each test	43/43	7–10 days	–	0.07	Only the digit span test was worse in the ≥35 °C group
1996					4–6 weeks	–	NS	
Grigore [35]	5	28 °C vs. 36 °C	>1 SD	110/117	6 weeks	39.3/39.1	0.99	No difference was observed
2001								
Nathan [36]	11	After rewarming 34 °C vs. 37 °C	>0.5 SD	111/112	1 week	48/62	0.048	34 °C was better
2001					3 months	–		Grooved pegboard test was better in 34 °C group
Nathan [37]	11	After rewarming 34 °C vs. 37 °C	>1 SD	66/65	1 week	46/32	0.045	34 °C was better
2007					5 years	44/42	0.781	Lower NTs scores in 1 week associated with those in 5 years
Grigore [38]	5	Slower rewarming vs. conventional rewarming	>1 SD	50/79	6 weeks	–	0.047	Slow rewarming affected NT scores
2002								
Boodhwani [39]	8	During and after CPB 34 °C vs. 37 °C	>1 SD	133/134	1 week	49/45	0.49	No difference was observed
2007					3 months	4/8	0.28	

(continued)

Table 5.2 (continued)

Author / Year	Number of tests	CPB management	Definition of POCD	Number of cases	Timing of evaluation	Development of POCD (%)	*P*-value	Comment
Acid base, perfusion, hematocrit, and blood glucose								
Gold [40]	11	PP during CPB, High (80–100 mmHg) vs. Low (50–60 mmHg)	Author determined the abnormal values in each test	112/113	1 week	–	–	No difference was observed. Only the finger tapping test was better in the high pressure group
1995					6 weeks	11/12	–	
Murkin [41]	4	α vs. pH-stat, pulsatile vs. no pulsatile	>20%	79/79	1 week	83/86	NS	
1995					2 months	27/44	0.047	α-stat was better when CPB time ≥90 min
Patel [42]	10	α-stat vs. pH-stat	>1 SD	35/35	6 weeks	20/49	0.02	α-stat was better
1996			Test number ≥3					
Mathew [43]	5	Hematocrit ≥27% vs. 15–18%	>1 SD	43/42	6 weeks	37.5/42.5	0.65	No difference was observed, but hemodilution and age were risk factors for POCD
2007								
Butterworth [44]	11	Blood glucose control (insulin) <100 mg/dL vs. non control	> 20%	188/193	4–8 days · 3–6 weeks	65/63 · 21/22	NS	No difference was observed
2005					5.5–6.5 months	13/18	NS	
Puskas [45]	5	Impact of hyperglycemia (≥200 mg/dL) on POCD in DM vs. non DM patients	>1 SD	145/380	6 weeks	38/41(DM)	0.81	Hyperglycemia was associated with the development of POCD in non-DM patients
2007						40/21(non DM)	0.017	

Filter and circuit								
Whitaker [46]	9	Leucocyte-depleting arterial line filter vs. other two conventional filters	*Z*-score	82/73+37	6–8 weeks	1.98/0.84 (*Z*-score)	0.07	Leucocyte-depleting arterial line filter was effective
2004			>1 SD			7.8/5.6	0.18	
Gerriets [47]	13	Intraaortic vs. dynamic bubble trap filters vs. conventional one	*Z*-score	38/47/41	3 months	–	–	Dynamic bubble trap filter was effective with fewer microemboli present and better NT scores
2010						–	–	
Heyer [48]	4	Heparin vs. non-heparin CBP circuits	Compared the total change score	26/35	5 days		0.04	Smaller decreases in NT scores in the heparin-bound CPB circuit was observed with low C3a concentration
2002					6 weeks		0.62	
Others								
Borger [49]	10	Decreasing the procedure during CPB by perfusionists	> 20%	42/41	3 months	50/34	0.18	No difference was observed
2001			> 2 tests					
Stygall [50]	9	Single cross clamp with cardioplegia vs. intermittent ventricular fibrillation	Compared the change rate in scores	82/95	1 day		NS	No difference was observed
2009					Discharge			

POCD postoperative cognitive dysfunction, *CPB* cardiopulmonary bypass, *ONCAB* on-pump coronary artery bypass grafting surgery, *NT* neuropsychological test, *SD* standard deviation, *PP* perfusion pressure, *DM* diabetes mellitus, *C3a* complement 3a the scattering of emboli is less frequent. However, the pH-stat strategy had a lower risk of postoperative neurodevelopmental impairment in pediatric cardiac surgery with circulatory arrest. This appears to be because in pediatric cardiac surgery, which is associated with fewer amounts of emboli, the brain is cooled more effectively by the blood vessels dilated by CO_2 load in the pH-stat strategy [51].

Perfusion pressure during CPB and effect of pulsatile flow on POCD have been investigated. Less frequent cerebral infarction was reported when perfusion pressure during CPB was maintained at as high as 80–100 mmHg rather than at 50–60 mmHg, but it is unclear whether these different perfusion pressure levels affect POCD [40]. A recent study showed that there are cases whose lower limit in cerebral blood flow autoregulation is set fairly higher than expected previously during CPB [52], and therefore further study is needed to elucidate proper perfusion pressure during CPB. It is also unclear whether pulsatile flow is effective for improving cerebral perfusion during CPB and can reduce the development of POCD [40].

The reduction in NT scores was shown to be suppressed when intraoperative hematocrit levels were maintained at ≥27% [43]. The high levels of blood glucose ≥200 mg/dL during ONCAB exacerbated the incidence rate of POCD in nondiabetic patients [45], but the effect of active maintenance of blood glucose levels <100 mg/dL by insulin administration on reducing the development of POCD was not observed [44].

Some studies attempted to modify filters and circuits used for CPB management. The use of leukocyte-depleting arterial line filters or dynamic bubble trap filters reduced the scattering of microemboli to the brain and thus decreased the incidence rate of POCD to a certain degree [46, 47]. In addition, the incidence rate of POCD was somewhat reduced by the use of a heparin-bonded CPB circuit that suppresses the activation of complement C3a [48]. Furthermore, ONCAB under ventricular fibrillation has been used to avoid cross-clamp cardioplegic arrest, but this procedure's efficacy for reducing in development of POCD was not observed [50].

Either way, all the studies showing the suppression of POCD by arranging the CPB management evaluated efficacy up to 2 months only (Table 5.2), and therefore the long-term efficacy is currently unknown.

5.3.4 Drug Administration During ONCAB and Its Effect on POCD

Among the studies that have investigated whether drug administration during ONCAB can reduce the incidence rate of POCD (Table 5.3) [53–64], some verified such efficacy using lidocaine because it is easy to use in ONCAB [54–56] (one study concerned valvular surgery [53]). Although early reports showed a reduction in the incidence rate of POCD [53, 54], long-term observation did not reveal efficacy [55, 56].

As for other drugs, because cardiovascular surgery including ONCAB has a high risk of cerebral infarction, drugs that had been effective in basic research using a cerebral infarction model were tested in clinical studies. Monosialotetrahexosyl ganglioside (GM1), an inhibitor of protein kinase C, plays a role in cell repair through the activation of Na^+/K^+ ATPase and adenylate cyclase, and the neuroprotective function of GM1 has been shown in basic studies. However, its effect on POCD in ONCAB was investigated in a preliminary study only, with no clear results [57]. In addition, the incidence rate of POCD did not reduce significantly in other studies using the antioxidant pegorgotein [59], the $GABA_A$ antagonist clomethazole [60], or the antiplatelet-activating factor lexipafant [61] and pexelizumab, a monoclonal antibody to C5 complement component [63]. Postmenopausal women often have the complication of cerebral infarction, probably because of the reduced levels of estrogen, which results in the elevation of cholesterol, especially low-density lipoprotein. The trial study was performed to administer 17-estradiol in postmenopausal women during ONCAB. However, it was not only ineffective but it worsened NT scores [64].

It was reported that the administration of remacemide, which is an NMDA antagonist and is used as an anticonvulsant [65], improved some NT scores [58], but no additional studies have been reported. In addition, the administration of aprotinin was shown to be beneficial for POCD, but the use of the drug was terminated in 2007 due to exacerbation of the drug-related mortality rate [62].

As indicated above, no drugs are currently capable of reducing the ONCAB-related incidence rate of POCD. However, as mentioned previously, the involvement of perioperative inflammatory responses is currently under investigation as the primary cause of POCD in basic research studies [28]. Further study is warranted to try to suppress the brain inflammation for reducing the development of POCD.

Table 5.3 The effect of drug administration on development of POCD in ONCAB

Author Year	Number of tests	Drug	Definition of POCD	Number of cases	Timing of evaluation	Development of POCD (%)	*P*-value	Comment
Lidcaine								
Mitchell [53]	6	1 mg/kg bolus followed by continuous infusion for 48 h (valvular surgery)	≥2 SD	25/24	10 days · 10 weeks	40/75 · 46/75	<0.025–0.05	Lidocaine was effective
1999				26/24 · 25/23	6 months	28/48	NS	
Wang [54]	6	1.5 mg/kg bolus and 4 mg/min intraoperatively	>1 SD	43/45	9 days	18.6/40.0	0.028	Lidocaine was effective
2002			≥2-test					
Mitchell [55]	7	1 mg/kg bolus, 2 mg/kg 2 h	>1 SD	59/59	10 weeks	45.8/40.7	0.577	No difference was observed
2009		1 mg/kg 12 h (including valvular surgery)		54/53	25 weeks	35.2/37.7	0.71	
Mathew [56]	5	1 mg/kg bolus, 4 mg/min for 1 h	>1 SD	88/94	6 weeks	45.5/45.7	0.97	No difference was observed
2009		2 mg/min for 1 h, 1 mg/min 46 h			1 year	40.0/51.7	0.185	
Other drugs								
Grieco [57]		Monosialotetrahexosyl ganglioside 300 mg 1 day before surgery and on the day	≥2 SD	18/11	1 week	77.8/72.8	NS	
1996				16/8	6 months	29.4/25	NS	No difference was observed
Arrowsmith [58]	10	Remacemide (NMDA antagonist) for 4 days before surgery and 5 days after surgery (150 mg 4 times/days)	Z-score	87/84	1 week	–		Some tests and total Z-scores were better in the treatment group
1998					8 weeks	–	0.028	

Butterworth [59]		Pegorgotein (anti-oxidant agent) 2000 or 5000 IU/kg IV before 6–18 h aorta clamp	≥20%	22/23/22	5–7 days	75/86/85	0.7	No difference was observed
1999				High/low/placebo	4–6 weeks	35/20/22	0.56	No difference was observed
Kong [60]	8	Clomethazole ($GABA_A$ agonist) loading dose 1.8 mg, 0.8 mg/h	> 20%	110/109	4–7 weeks	–	0.27–0.39	No difference was observed
2002			*Z*-score					
Taggart [61]	10	Lexipafant (anti-platelet activating factor),	Numbers of	46/45/40	Discharge	1.52/1.14/0.87	0.05	Drug had no effect or even worsened the NTs scores
2003		low (0.4 mg/kg) and high dose (4 mg) bolus continued for 24 h	the test (> 20%)	High/low/placebo	3 months	0.52/0.49/0.48	0.9	
Harmon [62]	6	Aprotinin, loading dose 2×10^6 KIU CPB 2×10^6 KIU, 5×10^5/h KIU during surgery	Reliable change index	17/18	4 days	58/94	0.01	A protinin was effective
2004					6 weeks	23/55	0.05	
Mathew [63]	5	Pexelizumab (monoclonal antibody to C5) 2 mg/kg bolus ± 0.05 mg/h	≥10%	238/245/239	4 days	48/57/46	0.07	Only the visual spatial domain was preserved in the treatment group
2004				bolus+cont/bolus/placebo	30 days	35/33/34	1	
Hogue [64]	7	17 -estradiol patch 1 day before surgery and 0.08 ng/kg/min	>1 SD	86/88 (+valvular surgery)	4–6 weeks	22/21	0.45	No difference was observed, but some scores worsened in the treatment group
2007			≥2-test	woman	6 months	23/15	0.82	

POCD postoperative cognitive dysfunction, *ONCAB* on-pump coronary artery bypass grafting surgery, *SD* standard deviation, *NS* not significant, *NMDA* *N*-methyl-D-aspartate, *GABA* γ-aminobutyric acid, *CPB* cardiopulmonary bypass, *cont* continuously

5.4 Development of POCD in ONCAB and OPCAB

We have so far explained the effect of ONCAB (with CPB) on POCD. To reveal the effect of CPB on POCD, the incidence rate of POCD in OPCAB (without CPB) was investigated in 26 studies, including 3 meta-analyses (Table 5.4) [66–91]. Eight of the studies reported a reduction in the incidence rate of POCD in OPCAB [66, 68, 72–74, 80–82], and none showed an increase in the incidence rate of it in OPCAB when compared to ONCAB. Most of the studies showing the superiority of OPCAB to ONCAB were characterized by the evaluation of POCD at the time of hospital discharge or 1 week to 6 months after surgery. The superiority of OPCAB was not observed in studies with a longer evaluation period. This suggests that compared with ONCAB, there is a possibility that higher brain cognition is maintained better for 6 months after OPCAB.

It is currently unclear why NT scores do not differ significantly between the two surgical procedures after 6 months, but the aging of patients is thought to adversely affect the NT scores.

5.5 Types of Treatment for Coronary Artery Disease and Change in Cognitive Function

To elucidate the effect of surgery itself on POCD in patients with a complication associated with coronary artery disease, some studies compared patients with coronary artery disease who had undergone ONCAB, OPCAB, PCI, or FCA (Table 5.5, top rows) [92–101]. By focusing on this point early on, Blumenthal et al. [92] showed that the prevalence of POCD at the time of hospital discharge was higher in the ONCAB group than in the PCI group [92]. However, only one other study showed the inferiority of ONCAB as compaired with PCI using NTs scores at 3 postoperative weeks [100]. Selnes et al. [94–98] performed a series of studies to investigate the incidence rate of POCD during a follow-up observation period of 3 months to 6 years in the ONCAB, OPCAB, PCI and FCA groups, using the *Z*-scores calculated based on the FCA or control people without coronary artery disease. Their findings showed that in the ONCAB, OPCAB, PCI, and FCA groups, the negative values of *Z*-scores were observed in all group preoperatively. *Z*-scores increased from 3 month to 1 year postoperatively but decreased from that point forward, with no significant intergroup difference. This result suggests that NT scores in the ONCAB group transitioned similarly, with no clear difference, to those in the OPCAB, PCI and FCA groups.

Observed no differences of NT scores changes along with passage of time between ONCAB and other treatment groups differ from the studies that we listed up in chapter 5.4 and Table 5.4, showing the inferiority of ONCAB for development of POCD. This is because no comparison study is conducted to show the differences of NT scores changes between the ONCAB, OPCAB, PCI and FCA in early postoperative period (<3 month). Assuming that the findings from early studies comparing the cognition between ONCAB and PCI are correct [92, 100], NT scores in ONCAB may be worse as compared with OPCAB, PCI and FCA around the time of hospital discharge or within 3 months of surgery.

Table 5.4 Development of POCD between ONCAB and OPCAB

Author Year	Number of tests	Definition of POCD	Timing of evaluation	ONCAB/ OPCAB cases	Development of POCD (%)	*P*-value	Comment
Diegeler [66]	2	Changes in scores	1 week	20/20	90/0	<0.01	Association between microemboli and declined score in ONCAB was observed
2000							
Lloyd [67]	7	Declined test numbers	1 year	30/30	2.19/2.13	0.9	Higher S100β protein was observed in OPCAB
2000							
Zamvar [68]	9	>1 SD scores	1 week	30/30	66/27	<0.01	OPCAB was better
2002		≥2-test	10 weeks		40/10	0.02	
Stroobant [69]	7	≥20%, 2-test	6 days	30/19	57/63	0.65	No difference was observed
2002			6 months	22/13	18/0	0.1	Higher score was observed in one NT in OPCAB
Lee [70]	9	≥20%, 20% test	2 weeks	29/29	15.4/16.1	NS	MIR detected the CBF reduction in ONCAB
2003			1 year	27/26	14.8/18.5	NS	Two NT scores were better in OPCAB
Lund [71]	10	≥20%, 2-test	3 months	52/54	23.1/20.4	0.74	Association between preoperative MRI abnormality and POCD was observed in ONCAB
2005			1 year	52/54	23.1/24.1	0.9	
Cheng [72]	37 references	Meta-analysis	1 month	–	51/40	0.3	No difference was observed
2005			2–6 months · 1 year	–	32/20 · 31/27	0.01 · 0.7	OPCAB was better
Takagi [73]	8 references	Meta-analysis	< 2 weeks	–	–	0.1935	
2007			1–3 months · 6–12 months	–	–	0.0162 · 0.8127	OPCAB was better

(continued)

Table 5.4 (continued)

Author Year	Number of tests	Definition of POCD	Timing of evaluation	ONCAB/ OPCAB cases	Development of POCD (%)	*P*-value	Comment
Al-Ruzzeh [74]	13	Changes in scores	6 weeks	79/80	–	<0.01	Scores in 3 NTs were better in OPCAB
2006			3 months · 6 months	76/75 · 72/73	–	<0.05	Scores in 2 NTs were better in OPCAB
Ernest [75]	11	>1.5 SD scores of published normal value	2 months	31/46	–	NS	
2006			6 months	32/47	–	NS	One NT was better in OPCAB
Van Dijk [76]	11	≥20%	3 months	120/128	29/21	0.15	Better improvement of NT scores was observed in OPCAB
2002			1 year	122/130	33.6/30.8	0.69	
van Dijk [77]		≥20%	5 years	117/123	50.4/50.4	>0.99	No difference was observed
2007							
Hammon [78]	11	≥20%	3–7 days	Single clamp 102/	60/60/70	0.439	No difference was observed
2006		≥2-test	3–6 weeks	Multi clamp 68/ OPCAB 68	32/51/39	0.325–0.485	
Jensen [79]	7	≥2-test	3 months	51/54	9.8/7.4	0.74	No difference was observed in three different analyses
2006		≥20% · Z-score			23.5/20.4 · 21.6/26	0.81 · 0.65	
Motallebzadeh [80]	7	Score differences	Discharge	104/108	–	0.01	
2007			6 weeks · 6 months	91/87 · 84/84	–	0.09 · 1	
Baba [81]	4	≥20%, 2-test	1 week	129/89	22.5/11.2	0.024	OPCAB was better
2007							

Yin [82]	5	>1 SD, 2-test	1 week	20/20	–	<0.05	Three NTs scores were worse in ONCAB than OPCAB
2007					–		
Hernandes [83]	19	≥20%	4 days	102/99	61.8/51.5	NS	One or two tests score were worse in OPCAB
2007		≥20% test	6 months		47.1/44.4	NS	
Marasco [84]	5	Meta-analysis	≤ 3 months	–	–	–	Better improvement in trail making test was shown in OPCAB
2008	8 references		≥6 months	–	–	–	
Jensen [85]	7	≥2-test	1 year	43/47	9.3/19.2	0.18	No difference was observed in three different analyses
2008		≥20% · *Z*-score			11.6/12.8 · 27.9/29.8	0.87 · 0.84	
Tully [86]	7	Comparing the scores	6 days	35/30	–	NS	No difference was observed
2008			6 months	31/28	–	NS	
Liu [87]	9	*Z*-score	1 week	59/168/C75	55.2/47.0	0.283	No difference was observed
2009			3 months		6.4/13.1	0.214	
Shroyer [88]	10	*Z*-score	1 year	581/575	0.17/0.19 (*Z*-score)		Only clock-drawing test was better in OPCAB
2009							
Kozora [89]	10	≥1 SD, 20% tests	1 year	581/575	12/13.2	0.595	No difference was observed
2010							
Sousa Uva [90]	8	*Z*-score	5 weeks	41/46/32C	–	–	Digit symbol was worse in ONCAB
2010							
Kennedy [91]	7	Meta-analysis	≤3 months	–	–	0.21–0.78	No difference was observed
2013	13 references		6–12 months	–	–	0.09–0.93	

POCD postoperative cognitive dysfunction, *ONCAB* on-pump coronary artery bypass grafting surgery, *OPCAB* off-pump CABG, *SD* standard deviation, *NT* neuropsychological test, *C* control

Table 5.5 Types of treatment for coronary artery disease and change in cognitive function

Author Year	Number of tests	Comparison	Definition of POCD	Timing of evaluation	Number of cases	Development of POCD (%)	*P*-value	Comment
ONCAB and other CAD								
Blumenthal [92]	5	ONCAB/PCI/ Valve	Score changes	Discharge	20/8/11	–	0.04	One NT score declined in ONCAB and valvular surgery, with no changes in the PCI group
1991								
Hlatky [93]	5	ONCAB/PCI	Scores changes	5 years	61/64	–	0.58	No difference was observed
1997								
Selnes [94]	16	ONCAB/FCA	*Z*-score	3 months	114/83	–	NS	No difference was observed
2003				1 year	116/77	–	NS	
Selnes [95]	16	ONCAB/FCA	*Z*-score	3 months	140/92	–	NS	*Z*-scores improved over 3 years
2005				1 year	121/83	–	NS	
				3 years	72/57	–	NS	
Selnes [96]	9	ONCAB/FCA	*Z*-score	6 years	96/61	–	NS	No difference was observed
2008								
Selnes [97]	16	ONCAB/ OPCAB/FCA/C	*Z*-score	3 months	121/54/91/65	–		From 1 year to 3 years, some NT scores worsened in the OPCAB and FCA group
2007				1 year	124/55/91/67	–		
				3 years	74/33/66/55	–		No significant differences were observed in the CAG group
Selnes [98]	6	ONCAB/ OPCAB/FCA/C	*Z*-score	6 years	96/43/67/60	–	NS	NTs scores were lower and declined in the CAG group
2009						–		
Währborg [99]	5	ONCAB/PCI	1 SD	6 months	64/71	–	0.22–1	No difference was observed
2004				1 year	64/66	–	0.23–0.68	

Rosengart [100]	14	ONCAB/PCI/C	>1 SD of normal published value or C reliable change indices	3 weeks	35/42/44	–	0.04	Only 1 NT score was worsened in ONCAB in 3 weeks
2006				4 months		–		
Sweet [101]	14	ONCAB/PCI/C	≥1.645 (Z-score)	3 weeks	39/42/44	–		7 and 3 NT scores worsened in 3 weeks and 1 year in CAG
2008				4 months	33/38/42	–		
				1 year	31/40/42	–		
ONCAB and other operation								
Vingerhoets [102]	11	Cardiac surgery vs. other major vascular or thoracic surgery	>1 SD, ≥ 2-test	7–8 days	91	45/40	NS	
1997				6 months		2016/12/21	NS	No difference was observed
Fearn [103]	16	ONCAB/ Urology	Reaction time	1 week	64/19	10/5 (declined test)	Significant	Low CO_2R by TCD and low perfusion pressure were risk factors
2001				2 months		2016/10/03	Significant	
				6 months		9/–		
Sugiyama [104]	3	ONCAB/ valvular surgery/vascular surgery	≥20%	10–14 days	65/37/24	46/43/38	NS	More patients with hypertension, DM, or hyperlipidemia were involved in the vascular group
2002								

POCD postoperative cognitive dysfunction, *ONCAB* on-pump coronary artery bypass grafting surgery, *PCI* percutaneous coronary intervention, *OPCAB* off-pump ONCAB, *C* control, *d* day, *w* week, *m* month, *NT* neuropsychological test, *ND* no difference, *FCA* follow-up coronary artery disease, *SD* standard deviation, *CAD* coronary artery disease group (ONCAB + OPCAB + FCA), *CO_2R* CO_2 response, *TCD* transcranial Doppler

5.6 Comparison of POCD Between ONCAB and Noncardiac Surgery

Only a very limited number of studies compared the incidence rate of POCD between ONCAB and noncardiac surgery [102–104] (Table 5.5, lower rows). Up to 2 months after surgery, the prevalence of POCD was overwhelmingly higher in ONCAB than in urological surgery [103], but the incidence rate was similar to that in thoracic or vascular surgery [102, 104]. However, preexisting complications were not investigated or standardized in the latter two studies [102, 104]. Therefore, the difference in the incidence rate of POCD between ONCAB and noncardiac surgery has not been fully elucidated.

5.7 Valvular Surgery and POCD

Compared with ONCAB, valvular surgery is associated with a high risk of scattering micoremboli to the brain during the open-heart surgical procedure, potentially inducing POCD. In Japan, the number of patients undergoing valvular surgery in recent years has been increasing due to the expansion of surgical indications to elderly individuals [2] and to the clinical application of transcatheter aortic valve implantation (TAVI). For this reason, it is more valuable to investigate the incidence rate of POCD in valvular surgery today. Representative studies are shown in Table 5.6 [105–117].

Previously, five studies compared the incidence rate of POCD between ONCAB and valvular surgery [105–109]. In a small sample size study of 22 patients, the incidence rate of POCD within 1 week of surgery was higher in patients who underwent ONCAB plus valvular surgery (POCD, 50%) than those who underwent ONCAB only (5%) [109]. In another study using brainstem auditory evoked potentials, the latency of event-related potential (P300) remained prolonged for 4 months only after valvular surgery [108]. However, no other study showed a clear difference.

Other studies of valvular surgery compared biological and mechanical valves in aortic valve replacement [110] and valve plasty and valve replacement in mitral valve surgery [111]. They revealed that the group of patients who had undergone the replacement of the aortic valve with a biological valve or mitral valve replacement had a high proportion of elderly individuals and a high incidence rate of POCD [110, 111].

The effect of robotic surgery and TAVI on POCD was also investigated. Compared with conventional surgery, robotic surgery may preserve brain function up to 1 week

Table 5.6 Comparison of the development of POCD in valvular surgery

Author Year	Number of tests	Comparison	Definition of POCD	Timing of evaluation	Number of cases	Development of POCD (%)	*P*-value	Comment
ONCAB vs. valuvular surgery								
Braekken [105]	15	ONCAB/valvular surgery	≥1 SD	5 days	/21	67	–	Association between microemboli and POCD was observed in valvular surgery
1998				2 months	14/26	14/23	0.06	
Andrew [106]	7	ONCAB/valvular surgery/C	Reliable change index	1 week	59/50/C56	50/50	–	Some NT scores were worse in valvular surgery in 6 months
2001			≥2 tests	6 months	44/30/C56	27/40	–	
Ebert [107]	6	ONCAB/Valvular surgery	>1.5 SD	2–3 days	42/42	57/71	0.172	No difference was observed
2001				1 week		36/19	0.087	
Zimpfer [108]	2	ONCAB/Valvular surgery (AVR)	Direct comparison of score and latency	1 week	53/29	–	0.607	Latency of P300 potential was prolonged in 1 week in both groups
2002				4 months		–	0.032	Its latency was still worsened in valvular surgery
Hudetz [109]	10	ONCAB/valvular surgery ± ONCAB/C	Z-score	1 week	22/22	5/50	<0.01	Development of delirium was a risk factor for POCD
2011			>1.5 SD					

(continued)

Table 5.6 (continued)

Author / Year	Number of tests	Comparison	Definition of POCD	Timing of evaluation	Number of cases	Development of POCD (%)	*P*-value	Comment
Valvular surgery								
Zimpfer [110]	2	AVR (biological/ mechanical valve)	>1 SD	1 week	29/53	52/45	0.114	Latency of P300 potential was prolonged in 1 week in both groups
2003				4 months		50/12	0.0001	Its latency was worse with a biological valve (higher age)
Grimm [111]	2	MVP/MVR	Change in scores	1 week	20/20	–	–	Biological valve group with higher-age cases was worse
2003			and latency	4 months		–	0.024	Scores in Trail making A worsened in MVR
Knipp [112]	13	Valvular surgery	Numbers of NTs that	5 days	30	Five out of 11 NTs decreased	0.05	Fourteen patients developed a new lesion on MRI without association with cognitive impairment
2005			score was decreased	4 months		0	–	
Hong [113]	3	Valvular surgery	Decreased ≥20%	1 week	100	23%	–	Decrease in rSO_2 was not associated with POCD
2008			or MMSE ≥ 3 points					
Fakin [114]	3	AVR (biological valve) hypothermic vs. normothermic CPB		1 week	30/30	–	NS	Latency of P300 was prolonged until 4 months
2012				4 months		–	NS	No difference was observed between the groups
Ferrari [115]	4	Mitral valve plasty by port access	Reliable change index	Discharge	72	–	NS	Except trail making B test, no significant impairment was observed
2014				3 months		–	NS	

Robotic surgery and TAVI								
Bruce [116]	7	Robotically/ conventional/ surgically C/ non-surgically C	≥20%, 20% tests	1 week	15/15/15/15	33.3/53.3/33.3	–	Low performance of cognition was observed in the conventional group, persisting until 1 week
2014				2 months		Not impaired	–	
Ghanem [117]	6	TAVI	>1 SD	3 days · 3 months	111	5.4 · 3.6	–	
2013				1 year · 2 years	86	3.6 · 3.6	–	

POCD postoperative cognitive dysfunction, *ONCAB* coronary artery bypass grafting surgery, *SD* standard deviation, *C* control, *NT* neuropsychological test, *AVR* aortic valve replacement, *MVP* mitral valve plasty, *MVR* mitral valve replacement, *MMSE* mini-mental state examination, *CPB* cardiopulmonary bypass, *NS* not significant, *TAVI* transcatheter aortic valve implantation

[116]. Interestingly, a study using minimally invasive TAVI showed that the incidence rate of POCD was as low as 5.4% despite a higher proportion of patients who were elderly or had serious conditions than that in conventional aortic valve replacement [117].

However, further study is needed to investigate the incidence of POCD in valvular surgery, by increasing the number of patients and NTs and the length of follow-up observation.

5.8 Major Vascular Surgery and POCD

As with valvular surgery, the number of patients undergoing major vascular surgery is on the rise in Japan [2]. CPB is especially complicated in major vascular surgery involving the aortic arch. In other words, because the distal anastomosis of artificial graft is performed using open distal anastomosis under circulatory arrest, the induction of deep hypothermia and selective perfusion to the brain are necessary to protect brain functions. For this, deep hypothermic circulatory arrest (DHCA), retrograde cerebral perfusion (RCP), or selective cerebral perfusion (SCP) is used. In major vascular surgery, which may limit the cerebral blood perfusion, it is extremely important to study the incidence rate of POCD, but it has not been investigated fully. This is partly because compared with ONCAB, the incidence rate of cerebral infarction that is more serious complication than POCD is high (around 10% in some studies), making the reduction of this serious complication the priority over the investigation of POCD. In addition, the development of seizure or delirium makes the assessment of POCD difficult. The assessment of POCD is more complicated by the long-term administration of sedatives for the continuous use of artificial ventilation.

Previous studies of POCD in major vascular surgery are shown in Table 5.7 [118–126]. Using DHCA (with no mention of body temperature), Ergin et al. [118] evaluated the prevalence of POCD at 1 and 6 weeks after surgery and showed that the incidence rate after 1 week was 31% and that the risk factors were arteriosclerotic aneurysm, surgery involving the aortic arch, and long duration of DHCA (>25 min). In a study using DHCA, RCP, and SCP, the prevalence of POCD was as high as 96% at 3–6 days after surgery but decreased to 9% after 2–3 weeks, with no significant difference in the incidence rate based on perfusion procedure [119]. Harrington et al. [121] compared the incidence rate of POCD between RCP and DHCA and found that the postoperative prevalence was high at 93% after RCP and 77% after DHCA at 6 weeks and was still 56% and 55% at 12 weeks, respectively. However, in another study, the prevalence of POCD was high at 16% in the RCP group compared with 1.5% in the DHCA group with a correlation between POCD and the duration of RCP [120]. When the incidence rate of POCD was compared between conventional CPB (valvular surgery and ONCAB), DHCA, and SCP, three tests showed postoperative exacerbation only in the SCP group, with a correlation between the duration of SCP and a decrease in the scores [126]. In addition, a study comparing the incidence rate

Table 5.7 POCD surgery

Author Year	Number of tests	Definition of POCD	Timing of evaluation	Number of cases CPB	DHCA	RCP	SCP	Development of POCD (%)	*P*-value	Comment
Ergin [118]	8	≥50%	1 week		71			31	–	Arteriosclerosis and DHCA time (>25 min) were risk factors
1999										
Svensson [119]	14	≥20%, 2 tests	3–6 days		10	10	10	96	NS	No difference was observed
2001			2–3 weeks					9	NS	Scores in DHCA group were better
Reich [120]	8	*Z*-score	16–121 days		69	25		1.5/16	0.0017	Risk factor was RCP time
2001										
Harrington [121]	7	≥20%, 2 tests	6 weeks		18	20		77/93	0.22	RCP showed no benefit
2003			3 months					56/55	0.93	
Özatik [122]	4	Changes in scores	1 week				22	0	–	No POCD was observed
2004			2 months					0		
Miyairi [123]	11	*Z*-score	2–3 weeks	28		46		–	–	Risk factor was RCP time (>60 min)
2005			4–6 months					–	NS	
Pacini [124]	17	Changes in scores	1 week	14			16	0	–	No difference was observed
2010			6 months					0	–	
Uysal [125]	7 (+daily life activities)	*Z*-score	≤ 6 years	207	67		26	–	–	Risk factor was DHCA time
2011										
Uysal [126]	14	*Z*-score	12–233 days	24	23		10	–	–	Risk factor was SCP time
2012										

POCD postoperative cognitive dysfunction, *CPB* cardiopulmonary bypass, *DHCA* deep hypothermic circulatory arrest, *RCP* retrograde cerebral perfusion, *SCP* selective cerebral perfusion of POCD in conventional CPB (ONCAB) and RCP revealed that postoperative test scores at 4–6 months were lower in the RCP group than those in the conventional CPB group when the duration of RCP was more than 60 min [123]. In a relatively large study using conventional CPB cases (ONCAB, valvular surgery, and ascending aortic replacement), DHCA, and SCP, the incidence rate of POCD was compared based on the activities of daily living of patients at 6 years after surgery. The results showed a correlation between the duration of DHCA and neural processing speed in the brain or memory impairment, with a decline in the reaction rate when the duration exceeded 21–24 min [125]. However, two studies reported that development of POCD was not observed unclear after SCP procedure [122, 124].

These findings suggest that in major vascular surgery, the incidence rate of POCD was higher in DHCA than in conventional CPB (ONCAB), and even when RCP was performed for intraoperative management, its efficacy would not be superior to the efficacy of DHCA. In addition, SCP may have a similar or even higher incidence rate of POCD than conventional CPB (ONCAB).

However, the investigations of POCD in major vascular surgery have problems. First, the number of patients is insufficient. Second, in some studies, an evaluating time point varied from a patient to a patient such as 12–233 days. Third, only a few studies investigated the incidence rate of POCD for more than 1 year, and therefore the long-term prevalence of POCD is unknown (Table 5.7). These issues need to be taken into consideration in further careful study.

5.9 Near-Infrared Spectroscopy Monitoring and POCD

Lastly, we would like to explain the relationship between POCD and intraoperative monitoring. In cardiac and major vascular surgery, near-infrared spectroscopy monitoring (NIRS) is used frequently to detect cerebral ischemia and prevent brain dysfunction. At least eight studies have investigated the association between POCD and a decrease in NIRS values [27, 113, 127–132]. In NIRS, regional cerebral oxygen saturation (rSO_2) measured by INVOS™ (Medtronic, USA) or tissue oxygen index (TOI) values measured by NIRO® (Hamamatsu Photonics, Japan) are commonly used for the assessment. These studies used actual values of 35–65% or 70–80% of the baseline value of rSO_2 or TOI as an alarm threshold value. However, these studies were conducted in ONCAB or valvular surgery, not in major vascular surgery. To date, five studies have reported the association between POCD and rSO_2 values [27, 128–132], whereas two studies have shown no association [113, 127] (Table 5.7). The exact cause for the conflicting results might have been the different criteria used for NT and POCD or different evaluation periods used among the studies.

The NIRS values have been shown to close to the values of SjO_2. However, the results showing the association between NIRS and POCD are in contrast to the results showing an unclear association between POCD and changes in SjO_2 which reflects blood circulation throughout the brain [12, 19]. It might be possible that NIRS captures hemodynamic changes in the frontal lobe that is associated with brain cognition.

Table 5.8 NIRS and POCD

Author Year	Number of tests	Type of surgery	Definition of POCD	Timing of evaluation	Cases	Development of POCD (%)	NIRS	Definition of abnormal value	Effectiveness of NIRS
Reents [127]	5	ONCAB	≥1 SD	6 days	47	34	INVOS™	$rSO_2 < 40$	No
2002							4100	$rSO_2 < 75\%$ baseline	
Yao [128]	2	ONCAB	≥20%, 1 SD	Discharge	101	18–24	INVOS™	$rSO_2 < 35$	Yes
2004		Valvular surgery					4100	$rSO_2 < 40$ 10 min	
Hong [113]	3	Valvular surgery	≥20%, or	1 week	100	23	INVOS™	$rSO_2 < 50$	No
2008			MMSE ≥ 3 points				5100	$rSO_2 < 80\%$ baseline	
Slater [129]	14	ONCAG	≥1 SD	3 months	240	60	INVOS™	$rSO_2 < 50$	Yes
2009							5100	AUC	
Shoen [27]	4	Cardiac	Change in scores	6 days	117		INVOS™	$rSO_2 < 50$	Yes
2011							5100		
Fudickar [130]	5	Cardiac	>20%, ≥2 tests	5 days	35	43	NIRO®	TOI < 65	Yes
2011							300		
de Tournay-Jette [131]	8	ONCAB+	≥1 SD, 2 tests	4–7 days	57	81	INVOS™	$rSO_2 < 50$	Yes
2011		OPCAB		1 month	61.0	39.0	4100	$rSO_2 < 70\%$ baseline	
Mohandas [132]	2	Cardiac	≥20%	1 week	100	–	Equanox	Active control to maintain	Yes
2013				3 months		–		>85% of baseline	MMSE scores were preserved

NIRS near-infrared spectroscopy, *POCD* postoperative cognitive dysfunction, *ONCAB* on-pump coronary artery bypass grafting surgery, *SD* standard deviation, rSO_2 regional cerebral oxygen saturation, *valve* valvular surgery, *MMSE* mini-mental state examination, *w* week, *m* month, *AUC* area under the curve, *TOI* tissue oxygen index, *OPCAB* off-pump CABG

Two of the studies reporting the association between NIRS and POCD investigated whether POCD improves when NIRS values were maintained by active management (keeping $PaCO_2$ high, mean blood pressure high, central venous pressure low, amount of CPB blood flow elevated, and hematocrit at ≥20%) [129, 132], with no consensus on the efficacy between the studies.

The number of studies reporting the association between POCD and a decrease in intraoperative NIRS values is increasing. However, these studies evaluated POCD for short periods of time. It is therefore necessary to investigate whether the active management of NIRS values improves prevalence of POCD over the long term (Table 5.8).

5.10 Conclusion

Various studies have been conducted to prevent the occurrence of POCD in ONCAB because, once POCD has developed, it can adversely affect patient prognosis. POCD may be prevented effectively by using the α-stat strategy during CPB and avoiding active re-warming from the end of CPB. At present, no drugs can alleviate POCD. However, it is thought that the difference in the incidence rate of POCD between ONCAB and PCI or FCA ceases to exist at or >6 months after surgery. This conversely suggests that the effect of surgery or CPB on POCD lasts for about 6 months after surgery.

Future challenges include the investigation of POCD in valvular surgery or major vascular surgery because the number of patients is expected to increase. However, because minimally invasive procedures such as TAVI and thoracic endovascular aortic repair may be applied in these surgeries, it will be interesting to ascertain whether minimally invasive procedures can reduce the incidence rate of POCD as in OPCAB and whether such beneficial effects last for the short or long term.

References

1. Arrowsmith JE, Grocott HP, Reves JG et al (2000) Central nervous system complications of cardiac surgery. Br J Anaesth 84:378–393
2. Amano J, Kuwano H, Yokomise H (2013) Thoracic and cardiovascular surgery in Japan during 2011: Annual report by The Japanese Association for Thoracic Surgery. Gen Thorac Cardiovasc Surg 61:578–607
3. Murkin JM, Newman SP, Stump DA et al (1995) Statement of consensus on assessment of neurobehavioral outcomes after cardiac surgery. Ann Thorac Surg 59:1289–1295
4. Rudolph JL, Schreiber KA, Culley DJ et al (2010) Measurement of post-operative cognitive dysfunction after cardiac surgery: a systematic review. Acta Anaesthesiol Scand 54:663–677
5. Mullges W, Babin-Ebell J, Reents W et al (2002) Cognitive performance after coronary artery bypass grafting: a follow-up study. Neurology 59:741–743
6. Dupuis G, Kennedy E, Lindquist R et al (2006) Coronary artery bypass graft surgery and cognitive performance. Am J Crit Care 15:471–478

7. Raymond PD, Hinton-Bayre AD, Radel M et al (2006) Assessment of statistical change criteria used to define significant change in neuropsychological test performance following cardiac surgery. Eur J Cardiothorac Surg 29:82–88
8. Browne SM, Halligan PW, Wade DT et al (1999) Cognitive performance after cardiac operation: implications of regression toward the mean. J Thorac Cardiovasc Surg 117:481–485
9. Kneebone AC, Luszcz MA, Baker RA et al (2005) A syndromal analysis of neuropsychological outcome following coronary artery bypass graft surgery. J Neurol Neurosurg Psychiatry 76:1121–1127
10. Walzer T, Herrmann M, Wallesch CW (1997) Neuropsychological disorders after coronary bypass surgery. J Neurol Neurosurg Psychiatry 62:644–648
11. Toner I, Taylor KM, Newman S et al (1998) Cerebral functional changes following cardiac surgery: Neuropsychological and EEG assessment. Eur J Cardiothorac Surg 13:13–20
12. Robson MJ, Alston RP, Deary IJ et al (2000) Cognition after coronary artery surgery is not related to postoperative jugular bulb oxyhemoglobin desaturation. Anesth Analg 91:1317–1326
13. Di Carlo A, Perna AM, Pantoni L et al (2001) Clinically relevant cognitive impairment after cardiac surgery: a 6-month follow-up study. J Neurol Sci 188:85–93
14. Millar K, Asbury AJ, Murray GD (2001) Pre-existing cognitive impairment as a factor influencing outcome after cardiac surgery. Br J Anaesth 86:63–67
15. Newman MF, Kirchner JL, Phillips-Bute B et al (2001) Longitudinal assessment of neurocognitive function after coronary-artery bypass surgery. N Engl J Med 344:395–402
16. Stygall J, Newman SP, Fitzgerald G et al (2003) Cognitive change 5 years after coronary artery bypass surgery. Health Psychol 22:579–586
17. Kruis RW, Vlasveld FA, Van Dijk D (2010) The (un)importance of cerebral microemboli. Semin Cardiothorac Vasc Anesth 14:111–118
18. Zimpfer D, Czerny M, Vogt F et al (2004) Neurocognitive deficit following coronary artery bypass grafting: a prospective study of surgical patients and nonsurgical controls. Ann Thorac Surg 78:513–519
19. Kadoi Y, Goto F (2006) Factors associated with postoperative cognitive dysfunction in patients undergoing cardiac surgery. Surg Today 36:1053–1057
20. Ramlawi B, Rudolph JL, Mieno S et al (2006) C-reactive protein and inflammatory response associated to neurocognitive decline following cardiac surgery. Surgery 140:221–226
21. Ramlawi B, Rudolph JL, Mieno S et al (2006) Serologic markers of brain injury and cognitive function after cardiopulmonary bypass. Ann Surg 244:593–601
22. Tardiff BE, Newman MF, Saunders AM et al (1997) Preliminary report of a genetic basis for cognitive decline after cardiac operations. The Neurologic Outcome Research Group of the Duke Heart Center. Ann Thorac Surg 64:715–720
23. Askar FZ, Cetin HY, Kumral E et al (2005) Apolipoprotein E epsilon4 allele and neurobehavioral status after on-pump coronary artery bypass grafting. J Card Surg 20:501–505
24. Tagarakis G, Tsolaki-Tagaraki F, Tsolaki M et al (2007) The role of SOAT-1 polymorphisms in cognitive decline and delirium after bypass heart surgery. Clin Res Cardiol 96:600–603
25. Silbert BS, Scott DA, Evered LA et al (2006) A comparison of the effect of high- and low-dose fentanyl on the incidence of postoperative cognitive dysfunction after coronary artery bypass surgery in the elderly. Anesthesiology 104:1137–1145
26. Hudetz JA, Iqbal Z, Gandhi SD et al (2009) Ketamine attenuates post-operative cognitive dysfunction after cardiac surgery. Acta Anaesthesiol Scand 53:864–872
27. Schoen J, Husemann L, Tiemeyer C et al (2011) Cognitive function after sevoflurane- vs propofol-based anaesthesia for on-pump cardiac surgery: a randomized controlled trial. Br J Anaesth 106:840–850
28. van Harten AE, Scheeren TW, Absalom AR (2012) A review of postoperative cognitive dysfunction and neuroinflammation associated with cardiac surgery and anaesthesia. Anaesthesia 67:280–293

29. Lamsa R, Helisalmi S, Herukka SK et al (2007) Study on the association between SOAT1 polymorphisms, Alzheimer's disease risk and the level of CSF biomarkers. Dement Geriatr Cogn Disord 24:146–150
30. Moller JT, Cluitmans P, Rasmussen LS et al (1998) Long-term postoperative cognitive dysfunction in the elderly ISPOCD1 study. ISPOCD investigators. International Study of Post-Operative Cognitive Dysfunction. Lancet 351:857–861
31. Rasmussen LS, Steentoft A, Rasmussen H et al (1999) Benzodiazepines and postoperative cognitive dysfunction in the elderly. ISPOCD Group. International Study of Postoperative Cognitive Dysfunction. Br J Anaesth 83:585–589
32. Hudetz JA, Patterson KM, Iqbal Z et al (2009) Ketamine attenuates delirium after cardiac surgery with cardiopulmonary bypass. J Cardiothorac Vasc Anesth 23:651–657
33. Regragui I, Birdi I, Izzat MB et al (1996) The effects of cardiopulmonary bypass temperature on neuropsychologic outcome after coronary artery operations: a prospective randomized trial. J Thorac Cardiovasc Surg 112:1036–1045
34. Mora CT, Henson MB, Weintraub WS et al (1996) The effect of temperature management during cardiopulmonary bypass on neurologic and neuropsychologic outcomes in patients undergoing coronary revascularization. J Thorac Cardiovasc Surg 112:514–522
35. Grigore AM, Mathew J, Grocott HP et al (2001) Prospective randomized trial of normothermic versus hypothermic cardiopulmonary bypass on cognitive function after coronary artery bypass graft surgery. Anesthesiology 95:1110–1119
36. Nathan HJ, Wells GA, Munson JL et al (2001) Neuroprotective effect of mild hypothermia in patients undergoing coronary artery surgery with cardiopulmonary bypass: a randomized trial. Circulation 104:I85–I91
37. Nathan HJ, Rodriguez R, Wozny D et al (2007) Neuroprotective effect of mild hypothermia in patients undergoing coronary artery surgery with cardiopulmonary bypass: five-year follow-up of a randomized trial. J Thorac Cardiovasc Surg 133:1206–1211
38. Grigore AM, Grocott HP, Mathew JP et al (2002) The rewarming rate and increased peak temperature alter neurocognitive outcome after cardiac surgery. Anesth Analg 94:4–10
39. Boodhwani M, Rubens F, Wozny D et al (2007) Effects of sustained mild hypothermia on neurocognitive function after coronary artery bypass surgery: a randomized, double-blind study. J Thorac Cardiovasc Surg 134:1443–1452
40. Gold JP, Charlson ME, Williams-Russo P et al (1995) Improvement of outcomes after coronary artery bypass. A randomized trial comparing intraoperative high versus low mean arterial pressure. J Thorac Cardiovasc Surg 110:1302–1314
41. Murkin JM, Martzke JS, Buchan AM et al (1995) A randomized study of the influence of perfusion technique and pH management strategy in 316 patients undergoing coronary artery bypass surgery. II. Neurologic and cognitive outcomes. J Thorac Cardiovasc Surg 110:349–362
42. Patel RL, Turtle MR, Chambers DJ et al (1996) Alpha-stat acid-base regulation during cardiopulmonary bypass improves neuropsychologic outcome in patients undergoing coronary artery bypass grafting. J Thorac Cardiovasc Surg 111:1267–1279
43. Mathew JP, Mackensen GB, Phillips-Bute B et al (2007) Effects of extreme hemodilution during cardiac surgery on cognitive function in the elderly. Anesthesiology 107:577–584
44. Butterworth J, Wagenknecht LE, Legault C et al (2005) Attempted control of hyperglycemia during cardiopulmonary bypass fails to improve neurologic or neurobehavioral outcomes in patients without diabetes mellitus undergoing coronary artery bypass grafting. J Thorac Cardiovasc Surg 130:1319
45. Puskas F, Grocott HP, White WD et al (2007) Intraoperative hyperglycemia and cognitive decline after CABG. Ann Thorac Surg 84:1467–1473
46. Whitaker DC, Newman SP, Stygall J et al (2004) The effect of leucocyte-depleting arterial line filters on cerebral microemboli and neuropsychological outcome following coronary artery bypass surgery. Eur J Cardiothorac Surg 25:267–274
47. Gerriets T, Schwarz N, Sammer G et al (2010) Protecting the brain from gaseous and solid micro-emboli during coronary artery bypass grafting: a randomized controlled trial. Eur Heart J 31:360–368

48. Heyer EJ, Lee KS, Manspeizer HE et al (2002) Heparin-bonded cardiopulmonary bypass circuits reduce cognitive dysfunction. J Cardiothorac Vasc Anesth 16:37–42
49. Borger MA, Peniston CM, Weisel RD et al (2001) Neuropsychologic impairment after coronary bypass surgery: effect of gaseous microemboli during perfusionist interventions. J Thorac Cardiovasc Surg 121:743–749
50. Stygall J, Suvarna S, Harrington J et al (2009) Effect on the brain of two techniques of myocardial protection. Asian Cardiovasc Thorac Ann 17:259–265
51. Abdul Aziz KA, Meduoye A (2010) Is pH-stat or alpha-stat the best technique to follow in patients undergoing deep hypothermic circulatory arrest? Interact Cardiovasc Thorac Surg 10:271–282
52. Brady K, Joshi B, Zweifel C et al (2010) Real-time continuous monitoring of cerebral blood flow autoregulation using near-infrared spectroscopy in patients undergoing cardiopulmonary bypass. Stroke 41:1951–1956
53. Mitchell SJ, Pellett O, Gorman DF (1999) Cerebral protection by lidocaine during cardiac operations. Ann Thorac Surg 67:1117–1124
54. Wang D, Wu X, Li J et al (2002) The effect of lidocaine on early postoperative cognitive dysfunction after coronary artery bypass surgery. Anesth Analg 95:1134–1141
55. Mitchell SJ, Merry AF, Frampton C et al (2009) Cerebral protection by lidocaine during cardiac operations: a follow-up study. Ann Thorac Surg 87:820–825
56. Mathew JP, Mackensen GB, Phillips-Bute B et al (2009) Randomized, double-blinded, placebo controlled study of neuroprotection with lidocaine in cardiac surgery. Stroke 40:880–887
57. Grieco G, d'Hollosy M, Culliford AT et al (1996) Evaluating neuroprotective agents for clinical anti-ischemic benefit using neurological and neuropsychological changes after cardiac surgery under cardiopulmonary bypass. Methodological strategies and results of a double-blind, placebo-controlled trial of GM1 ganglioside. Stroke 27:858–874
58. Arrowsmith JE, Harrison MJ, Newman SP et al (1998) Neuroprotection of the brain during cardiopulmonary bypass: a randomized trial of remacemide during coronary artery bypass in 171 patients. Stroke 29:2357–2362
59. Butterworth J, Legault C, Stump DA et al (1999) A randomized, blinded trial of the antioxidant pegorgotein: no reduction in neuropsychological deficits, inotropic drug support, or myocardial ischemia after coronary artery bypass surgery. J Cardiothorac Vasc Anesth 13:690–694
60. Kong RS, Butterworth J, Aveling W et al (2002) Clinical trial of the neuroprotectant clomethiazole in coronary artery bypass graft surgery: a randomized controlled trial. Anesthesiology 97:585–591
61. Taggart DP, Browne SM, Wade DT et al (2003) Neuroprotection during cardiac surgery: a randomised trial of a platelet activating factor antagonist. Heart 89:897–900
62. Harmon DC, Ghori KG, Eustace NP et al (2004) Aprotinin decreases the incidence of cognitive deficit following CABG and cardiopulmonary bypass: a pilot randomized controlled study. Can J Anaesth 51:1002–1009
63. Mathew JP, Shernan SK, White WD et al (2004) Preliminary report of the effects of complement suppression with pexelizumab on neurocognitive decline after coronary artery bypass graft surgery. Stroke 35:2335–2339
64. Hogue CW Jr, Freedland K, Hershey T et al (2007) Neurocognitive outcomes are not improved by 17beta-estradiol in postmenopausal women undergoing cardiac surgery. Stroke 38:2048–2054
65. Malek R, Borowicz KK, Kimber-Trojnar Z et al (2003) Remacemide--a novel potential antiepileptic drug. Pol J Pharmacol 55:691–698
66. Diegeler A, Hirsch R, Schneider F et al (2000) Neuromonitoring and neurocognitive outcome in off-pump versus conventional coronary bypass operation. Ann Thorac Surg 69:1162–1166
67. Lloyd CT, Ascione R, Underwood MJ et al (2000) Serum S-100 protein release and neuropsychologic outcome during coronary revascularization on the beating heart: a prospective randomized study. J Thorac Cardiovasc Surg 119:148–154
68. Zamvar VY, Khan NU, Madhavan A et al (2002) Clinical outcomes in coronary artery bypass graft surgery: comparison of off-pump and on-pump techniques. Heart Surg Forum 5:109–113
69. Stroobant N, Van Nooten G, Belleghem Y et al (2002) Short-term and long-term neurocognitive outcome in on-pump versus off-pump CABG. Eur J Cardiothorac Surg 22:559–564

70. Lee JD, Lee SJ, Tsushima WT et al (2003) Benefits of off-pump bypass on neurologic and clinical morbidity: a prospective randomized trial. Ann Thorac Surg 76:18–26
71. Lund C, Sundet K, Tennoe B et al (2005) Cerebral ischemic injury and cognitive impairment after off-pump and on-pump coronary artery bypass grafting surgery. Ann Thorac Surg 80:2126–2131
72. Cheng DC, Bainbridge D, Martin JE et al (2005) Does off-pump coronary artery bypass reduce mortality, morbidity, and resource utilization when compared with conventional coronary artery bypass? A meta-analysis of randomized trials. Anesthesiology 102:188–203
73. Takagi H, Tanabashi T, Kawai N et al (2007) Cognitive decline after off-pump versus on-pump coronary artery bypass graft surgery: meta-analysis of randomized controlled trials. J Thorac Cardiovasc Surg 134:512–513
74. Al-Ruzzeh S, George S, Bustami M et al (2006) Effect of off-pump coronary artery bypass surgery on clinical, angiographic, neurocognitive, and quality of life outcomes: randomised controlled trial. BMJ 332:1365
75. Ernest CS, Worcester MU, Tatoulis J et al (2006) Neurocognitive outcomes in off-pump versus on-pump bypass surgery: a randomized controlled trial. Ann Thorac Surg 81:2105–2114
76. Van Dijk D, Jansen EW, Hijman R et al (2002) Cognitive outcome after off-pump and on-pump coronary artery bypass graft surgery: a randomized trial. JAMA 287:1405–1412
77. van Dijk D, Spoor M, Hijman R et al (2007) Cognitive and cardiac outcomes 5 years after off-pump vs on-pump coronary artery bypass graft surgery. JAMA 297:701–708
78. Hammon JW, Stump DA, Butterworth JF et al (2006) Single crossclamp improves 6-month cognitive outcome in high-risk coronary bypass patients: the effect of reduced aortic manipulation. J Thorac Cardiovasc Surg 131:114–121
79. Jensen BO, Hughes P, Rasmussen LS et al (2006) Cognitive outcomes in elderly high-risk patients after off-pump versus conventional coronary artery bypass grafting: a randomized trial. Circulation 113:2790–2795
80. Motallebzadeh R, Bland JM, Markus HS et al (2007) Neurocognitive function and cerebral emboli: randomized study of on-pump versus off-pump coronary artery bypass surgery. Ann Thorac Surg 83:475–482
81. Baba T, Goto T, Maekawa K et al (2007) Early neuropsychological dysfunction in elderly high-risk patients after on-pump and off-pump coronary bypass surgery. J Anesth 21:452–458
82. Yin YQ, Luo AL, Guo XY et al (2007) Postoperative neuropsychological change and its underlying mechanism in patients undergoing coronary artery bypass grafting. Chin Med J 120:1951–1957
83. Hernandez F Jr, Brown JR, Likosky DS et al (2007) Neurocognitive outcomes of off-pump versus on-pump coronary artery bypass: a prospective randomized controlled trial. Ann Thorac Surg 84:1897–1903
84. Marasco SF, Sharwood LN, Abramson MJ (2008) No improvement in neurocognitive outcomes after off-pump versus on-pump coronary revascularisation: a meta-analysis. Eur J Cardiothorac Surg 33:961–970
85. Jensen BO, Rasmussen LS, Steinbruchel DA (2008) Cognitive outcomes in elderly high-risk patients 1 year after off-pump versus on-pump coronary artery bypass grafting. A randomized trial. Eur J Cardiothorac Surg 34:1016–1021
86. Tully PJ, Baker RA, Kneebone AC et al (2008) Neuropsychologic and quality-of-life outcomes after coronary artery bypass surgery with and without cardiopulmonary bypass: a prospective randomized trial. J Cardiothorac Vasc Anesth 22:515–521
87. Liu YH, Wang DX, Li LH et al (2009) The effects of cardiopulmonary bypass on the number of cerebral microemboli and the incidence of cognitive dysfunction after coronary artery bypass graft surgery. Anesth Analg 109:1013–1022
88. Shroyer AL, Grover FL, Hattler B et al (2009) On-pump versus off-pump coronary-artery bypass surgery. N Engl J Med 361:1827–1837
89. Kozora E, Kongs S, Collins JF et al (2010) Cognitive outcomes after on- versus off-pump coronary artery bypass surgery. Ann Thorac Surg 90:1134–1141
90. Sousa Uva M, Cavaco S, Oliveira AG et al (2010) Early graft patency after off-pump and on-pump coronary bypass surgery: a prospective randomized study. Eur Heart J 31:2492–2499

91. Kennedy ED, Choy KC, Alston RP et al (2013) Cognitive outcome after on- and off-pump coronary artery bypass grafting surgery: a systematic review and meta-analysis. J Cardiothorac Vasc Anesth 27:253–265
92. Blumenthal JA, Madden DJ, Burker EJ et al (1991) A preliminary study of the effects of cardiac procedures on cognitive performance. Int J Psychosom 38:13–16
93. Hlatky MA, Bacon C, Boothroyd D et al (1997) Cognitive function 5 years after randomization to coronary angioplasty or coronary artery bypass graft surgery. Circulation 96:II–11–15
94. Selnes OA, Grega MA, Borowicz LM Jr et al (2003) Cognitive changes with coronary artery disease: a prospective study of coronary artery bypass graft patients and nonsurgical controls. Ann Thorac Surg 75:1377–1386
95. Selnes OA, Grega MA, Borowicz LM et al (2005) Cognitive outcomes three years after coronary artery bypass surgery: a comparison of on-pump coronary artery bypass graft surgery and nonsurgical controls. Ann Thorac Surg 79:1201–1209
96. Selnes OA, Grega MA, Bailey MM et al (2008) Cognition 6 years after surgical or medical therapy for coronary artery disease. Ann Neurol 63:581–590
97. Selnes OA, Grega MA, Bailey MM et al (2007) Neurocognitive outcomes 3 years after coronary artery bypass graft surgery: a controlled study. Ann Thorac Surg 84:1885–1896
98. Selnes OA, Grega MA, Bailey MM et al (2009) Do management strategies for coronary artery disease influence 6-year cognitive outcomes? Ann Thorac Surg 88:445–454
99. Wahrborg P, Booth JE, Clayton T et al (2004) Neuropsychological outcome after percutaneous coronary intervention or coronary artery bypass grafting: results from the Stent or Surgery (SoS) Trial. Circulation 110:3411–3417
100. Rosengart TK, Sweet JJ, Finnin E et al (2006) Stable cognition after coronary artery bypass grafting: comparisons with percutaneous intervention and normal controls. Ann Thorac Surg 82:597–607
101. Sweet JJ, Finnin E, Wolfe PL et al (2008) Absence of cognitive decline one year after coronary bypass surgery: comparison to nonsurgical and healthy controls. Ann Thorac Surg 85:1571–1578
102. Vingerhoets G, Van Nooten G, Vermassen F et al (1997) Short-term and long-term neuropsychological consequences of cardiac surgery with extracorporeal circulation. Eur J Cardiothorac Surg 11:424–431
103. Fearn SJ, Pole R, Wesnes K et al (2001) Cerebral injury during cardiopulmonary bypass: emboli impair memory. J Thorac Cardiovasc Surg 121:1150–1160
104. Sugiyama N, Kawaguchi M, Yoshitani K et al (2002) The incidence and severity of cognitive decline after major noncardiac surgery: a comparison with that after cardiac surgery with cardiopulmonary bypass. J Anesth 16:261–264
105. Braekken SK, Reinvang I, Russell D et al (1998) Association between intraoperative cerebral microembolic signals and postoperative neuropsychological deficit: comparison between patients with cardiac valve replacement and patients with coronary artery bypass grafting. J Neurol Neurosurg Psychiatry 65:573–576
106. Andrew MJ, Baker RA, Bennetts J et al (2001) A comparison of neuropsychologic deficits after extracardiac and intracaradiac surgery. J Cardiothorac Vasc Anesth 15:9–14
107. Ebert AD, Walzer TA, Huth C et al (2001) Early neurobehavioral disorders after cardiac surgery: a comparative analysis of coronary artery bypass graft surgery and valve replacement. J Cardiothorac Vasc Anesth 15:15–19
108. Zimpfer D, Czerny M, Kilo J et al (2002) Cognitive deficit after aortic valve replacement. Ann Thorac Surg 74:407–412
109. Hudetz JA, Iqbal Z, Gandhi SD et al (2011) Postoperative delirium and short-term cognitive dysfunction occur more frequently in patients undergoing valve surgery with or without coronary artery bypass graft surgery compared with coronary artery bypass graft surgery alone: results of a pilot study. J Cardiothorac Vasc Anesth 25:811–816
110. Zimpfer D, Kilo J, Czerny M et al (2003) Neurocognitive deficit following aortic valve replacement with biological/mechanical prosthesis. Eur J Cardiothorac Surg 23:544–551
111. Grimm M, Zimpfer D, Czerny M et al (2003) Neurocognitive deficit following mitral valve surgery. Eur J Cardiothorac Surg 23:265–271

112. Knipp SC, Matatko N, Schlamann M et al (2005) Small ischemic brain lesions after cardiac valve replacement detected by diffusion-weighted magnetic resonance imaging: relation to neurocognitive function. Eur J Cardiothorac Surg 28:88–96
113. Hong SW, Shim JK, Choi YS et al (2008) Prediction of cognitive dysfunction and patients' outcome following valvular heart surgery and the role of cerebral oximetry. Eur J Cardiothorac Surg 33:560–565
114. Fakin R, Zimpfer D, Sodeck GH et al (2012) Influence of temperature management on neurocognitive function in biological aortic valve replacement. A prospective randomized trial. J Cardiovasc Surgery 53:107–112
115. Ferrari R, Vidotto G, Muzzolon C et al (2014) Neurocognitive deficit and quality of life after mitral valve repair. J Heart Valve Dis 23:72–78
116. Bruce KM, Yelland GW, Almeida AA et al (2014) Effects on cognition of conventional and robotically assisted cardiac valve operation. Ann Thorac Surg 97:48–55
117. Ghanem A, Kocurek J, Sinning JM et al (2013) Cognitive trajectory after transcatheter aortic valve implantation. Circ Cardiovasc Interv 6:615–624
118. Ergin MA, Uysal S, Reich DL et al (1999) Temporary neurological dysfunction after deep hypothermic circulatory arrest: a clinical marker of long-term functional deficit. Ann Thorac Surg 67:1887–1890
119. Svensson LG, Nadolny EM, Penney DL et al (2001) Prospective randomized neurocognitive and S-100 study of hypothermic circulatory arrest, retrograde brain perfusion, and antegrade brain perfusion for aortic arch operations. Ann Thorac Surg 71:1905–1912
120. Reich DL, Uysal S, Ergin MA et al (2001) Retrograde cerebral perfusion during thoracic aortic surgery and late neuropsychological dysfunction. Eur J Cardiothorac Surg 19:594–600
121. Harrington DK, Bonser M, Moss A et al (2003) Neuropsychometric outcome following aortic arch surgery: a prospective randomized trial of retrograde cerebral perfusion. J Thorac Cardiovasc Surg 126:638–644
122. Ozatik MA, Kucuker SA, Tuluce H et al (2004) Neurocognitive functions after aortic arch repair with right brachial artery perfusion. Ann Thorac Surg 78:591–595
123. Miyairi T, Takamoto S, Kotsuka Y et al (2005) Comparison of neurocognitive results after coronary artery bypass grafting and thoracic aortic surgery using retrograde cerebral perfusion. Eur J Cardiothorac Surg 28:97–103
124. Pacini D, Di Marco L, Leone A et al (2010) Cerebral functions and metabolism after antegrade selective cerebral perfusion in aortic arch surgery. Eur J Cardiothorac Surg 37:1322–1331
125. Uysal S, Mazzeffi M, Lin HM et al (2011) Internet-based assessment of postoperative neurocognitive function in cardiac and thoracic aortic surgery patients. J Thorac Cardiovasc Surg 141:777–781
126. Uysal S, Lin HM, Fischer GW et al (2012) Selective cerebral perfusion for thoracic aortic surgery: association with neurocognitive outcome. J Thorac Cardiovasc Surg 143:1205–1212
127. Reents W, Muellges W, Franke D et al (2002) Cerebral oxygen saturation assessed by near-infrared spectroscopy during coronary artery bypass grafting and early postoperative cognitive function. Ann Thorac Surg 74:109–114
128. Yao FS, Tseng CC, Ho CY et al (2004) Cerebral oxygen desaturation is associated with early postoperative neuropsychological dysfunction in patients undergoing cardiac surgery. J Cardiothorac Vasc Anesth 18:552–558
129. Slater JP, Guarino T, Stack J et al (2009) Cerebral oxygen desaturation predicts cognitive decline and longer hospital stay after cardiac surgery. Ann Thorac Surg 87:36–45
130. Fudickar A, Peters S, Stapelfeldt C et al (2011) Postoperative cognitive deficit after cardiopulmonary bypass with preserved cerebral oxygenation: a prospective observational pilot study. BMC Anesthesiol 11:7
131. de Tournay-Jette E, Dupuis G, Bherer L et al (2011) The relationship between cerebral oxygen saturation changes and postoperative cognitive dysfunction in elderly patients after coronary artery bypass graft surgery. J Cardiothorac Vasc Anesth 25:95–104
132. Mohandas BS, Jagadeesh AM, Vikram SB (2013) Impact of monitoring cerebral oxygen saturation on the outcome of patients undergoing open heart surgery. Ann Card Anaesth 16:102–106

Chapter 6
Present Clinical Status of Postoperative Cognitive Dysfunction Following Noncardiac Surgery

Tatsuo Horiuchi, Tomonori Takazawa, and Shigeru Saito

Abstract Postoperative cognitive dysfunction (POCD) after noncardiac surgery is less frequent than that after cardiac surgery. However, POCD after noncardiac surgery has become an important perioperative clinical issue particularly for geriatric surgical patients. In fact, it has been demonstrated that POCD is associated with increased mortality. Patients suffering from POCD usually complain of deterioration of memory as the initial symptom. Most patients do not notice that their symptoms may have been caused by the surgery, because they have no knowledge about POCD. For detecting POCD, it is necessary to perform several neurophysiological tests. Furthermore, physicians must be aware that a wide spectrum of cognitive functions, such as memory, attention, and information processing, are impaired in some of the patients. There is no established therapeutic protocol for POCD, although the risk factors of POCD have been identified. Hence, anesthesiologists and surgeons should have knowledge about the clinical status and risk factors of POCD so that they can preoperatively evaluate the risk of POCD in patients and prevent its occurrence.

Keywords Postoperative cognitive dysfunction • Noncardiac surgery • Mild cognitive impairment

6.1 Introduction

POCD is generally described as a postoperative decline in cognitive function as compared to the patient's preoperative cognitive status. Although this decline in cognitive function is usually subtle in nature and may be unrecognized by clinicians [1],

T. Horiuchi • T. Takazawa (✉) • S. Saito
Department of Anesthesiology, Gunma University Graduate School of Medicine,
3-39-22 Showa-Machi, Maebashi, Gunma 371-8511, Japan
e-mail: takazawt@gunma-u.ac.jp

Y. Morimoto (ed.), *Anesthesia and Neurotoxicity*,
DOI 10.1007/978-4-431-55624-4_6

POCD affects a wide variety of cognitive domains, such as attention, memory, executive function, and speed of information processing [2]. POCD was first reported by Bedford in 1955 [3] and, since then, many studies have been performed mainly to investigate POCD after cardiac surgery. However, POCD after noncardiac surgery has also been recently noted [4–8]. The reasons why POCD has been in the spotlight are as follows. Patients who have POCD at both hospital discharge and 3 months after surgery are more likely to die in the first year after surgery, suggesting that POCD is associated with increased mortality [5]. In addition, POCD is associated with the risk of premature exit from the workforce and dependence on social security [9]. These evidences suggest that POCD could affect not only patients but also their next of kin and colleagues, indicating that avoidance of POCD is an important public health issue. This chapter focuses principally on the present clinical status of POCD after noncardiac surgery. Moreover, we discuss the epidemiology, differential diagnosis, putative mechanisms, risk factors, and screening tools for POCD.

6.2 Epidemiology of POCD After Noncardiac Surgery

To date, numerous studies on POCD after noncardiac surgery have been conducted [4, 5, 8, 10–13]. Previously, there were several issues in the identification of POCD. For example, there was no consensus on the definition of POCD and the tests required for its detection. A change came in the mid-1990s when researchers started to define POCD as a decline in performance following surgery on at least two or three tests in a sensitive test battery [14]. Although the number of studies investigating POCD after noncardiac surgery has increased, reported incidences of POCD at 3 months after surgery still vary from 8% [8] to 53% [11]. This variance is likely to be caused by the methodological differences in determining patient characteristics, and the timing and type of neuropsychological tests used to detect POCD. The overall consensus is that POCD after noncardiac surgery seems to be less frequent than that after cardiac surgery.

6.3 Present Clinical Status of POCD

The most noticeable subjective symptoms of POCD are deficits in memory and a reduced ability to handle intellectual challenges [2, 15–17]. POCD itself is not life threatening, and the subtle differences in cognitive performance are extremely difficult to measure [18]. Thus, anesthesiologists and/or surgeons may not be aware of the presence of symptoms of POCD in the patients. In most cases, the patient has no knowledge about POCD. Even if the patient realizes the postoperative cognitive decline, they do not associate their symptoms with the surgery.

Cognitive functions such as perception, language processing, attention and memory functions, and abstract thinking are crucial for daily life activities, affecting

Table 6.1 Summary of the cognitive domains and relevant neuropsychological tests that can be used for investigating postoperative cognitive dysfunction

	Cognitive domain	Test
Memory	Working memory Encoding and retrieval of long-term memory	Digit span Verbal and visual recall and recognition
Attention	Mental flexibility Selective attention General	Trail making test Stroop test ECO attention, WMS-R
Information processing	Information processing Language processing Visuospatial processing	Substitution test

everyday tasks varying from driving and cooking to complex social interaction [17]. Patients suffering from POCD usually complain about deterioration of memory as the initial symptom. This is usually not apparent immediately after the surgery, and in many cases is not detected until the patient, family members, or colleagues notice that the patient is having difficulties with normal activities at home or work [19]. Patients often describe their dysfunction as memory loss, lack of concentration, or slowness in executive and abstract functions [17].

For objective tests to detect POCD, cognitive functions are often categorized into three domains, namely memory, attention, and information processing (Table 6.1). Past studies demonstrated that memory functions, especially visual and verbal recall, seem to be affected in the highest number of patients [6, 20]. Moreover, language and visuospatial processing decline in a relatively large percentage of patients after surgery, with up to 15% of patients experiencing a decline in performance [14]. In contrast, the attention domain is affected in a smaller percentage of patients. However, attention impairments have been consistently demonstrated in a number of tests and studies. In addition, concentration problems are frequently mentioned by patients after surgery [21–23]. Therefore, one may argue that cognitive complaints after surgery may not correlate well with objective measurements of POCD [14]. If this is true, researchers will have to reconsider methods to determine POCD.

6.4 Differential Diagnosis of POCD (Table 6.2)

Neurological disorders after surgery are classified into POCD, postoperative delirium (POD), and stroke (cerebral infarction) [18, 24]. In most cases, stroke can be diagnosed by imaging studies, such as computed tomography (CT) and magnetic resonance imaging (MRI). However, it is difficult to diagnose POCD and POD with these imaging studies. In addition, POD and POCD are often reported as being part of the same continuum of postoperative cognitive impairment [2]. Thus, knowledge about the epidemiology and clinical status of POD is essential to distinguish between POD and POCD. The key characteristics of POD are a change in mental status, characterized by reduced awareness of the environment and disturbance in

Table 6.2 Differential diagnosis of cerebral disorders after surgery

	Symptom	Diagnostic methods	Prognosis
POCD	Cognitive dysfunctions (attention, memory, executive function, and speed of information processing)	Comparisons of the pre- and postoperative results in multiple neurological tests	Recover in most cases
POD	Hallucinations, decline in cognition and attention and inappropriate behavior	Delirium scale (Nu-DESC, NEECHAM,CAM-ICU, etc.)	Usually respond to medical treatment
Stroke	Various symptoms including consciousness disorder, paralysis, aphasia, and agnosia	Brain imaging (CT, MRI, MRA)	Various (depend on the severity)

attention. This may be accompanied by other, more florid, perceptual symptoms (hallucinations) or cognitive symptoms, including disorientation or temporary memory dysfunction. The patient may express hypoactive, hyperactive, or mixed psychomotor behaviors [25]. POD develops in up to 56% of the patients (higher risk in elderly patients and after orthopedic surgery) [26]. Although POD is far from benign, patients with POD are more likely to demonstrate initial complete recovery as compared to other forms of delirium [27]. As mentioned above, POD and POCD show similar symptoms in many cases. However, the diagnostic tools for delirium are much more established than those for POCD. Therefore, it is not difficult to diagnose POD if physicians are aware of the fact that delirium can occur in patients after surgery.

6.5 Putative Mechanisms of POCD After Noncardiac Surgery

Many studies have suggested that inflammatory responses are associated with postoperative cognitive dysfunction [19, 28, 29]. Indeed, the levels of proinflammatory cytokines, such as IL-6, measured in cerebrospinal fluid were increased in postoperative patients [30, 31]. Preclinical studies demonstrated that a surgery-induced innate immune response triggered an IL-1β-mediated inflammatory process in the hippocampus, which underlies memory impairment [32, 33]. Recently, the role of astrocytes and microglia in cognitive impairment after surgery has been shown [34, 35]. For example, aged rats demonstrated significant deficits in memory and learning shortly after surgery, accompanied by activation of microglia and marked upregulation of TLR4 on microglia in the hippocampus [35]. Although several mechanisms that probably contribute to the development of POCD have been proposed, further studies are still required.

As mentioned above, a wide spectrum of cognitive functions are impaired in patients with POCD. In fact, the areas possibly involved in POCD include prefrontal, frontal, parietal, temporal, occipital, hippocampal, insular, cingulate, thalamic, and cerebellar regions. Even a single domain of cognitive function usually requires coordinated activation of several cerebellar regions. In other words, malfunction in a specific cerebellar region can impact multiple domains of cognitive function [14]. The hippocampus seems especially vulnerable to inflammation-mediated changes [36]. Consequently, preclinical studies have mainly focused on the role of inflammation in surgery-induced decline of hippocampal function [32, 33, 37, 38]. Although the hippocampus plays a significant role in long-term memory, the contribution of the hippocampus to other cognitive functions, including attention and information processing, seems to be modest [14]. Taken together, functional changes in the cerebellar region, rather than the hippocampus, after surgery require thorough investigation.

6.6 Risk Factors and Screening Tools of POCD

Increasing age, duration of anesthesia, low levels of education, a second operation, postoperative infections, and respiratory complications are reportedly risk factors for POCD [4]. In addition, cognitive functions were more profoundly impaired in patients with mild preoperative cognitive impairment (MCI) [39], metabolic syndrome [6], blood transfusion [40], and a small hippocampus [7]. These risk factors can be divided into two categories: preoperative cerebral vulnerabilities and incidents occurring during the perioperative period, which could affect cognitive function. Preoperative interviews may make it possible to screen patients who are at a high risk of POCD. In particular, screening cerebral vulnerabilities in patients before the surgery seems to be a good approach for avoiding POCD. We will now discuss how we can identify pre-existing cognitive dysfunction (i.e., MCI).

MCI is defined as impairment of one or more cognitive domains to a greater extent than would be expected for the person's age, but which does not yet interfere with their abilities of daily life. The prevalence of MCI in subjects over 65 years old is reportedly 23.5% [41]. Given that the elderly population is likely to increase, the number of patients with MCI is expected to increase in the future. Mini-Mental State Examination (MMSE) has been used in clinical studies on POCD to evaluate cognitive function [42–46]. However, MMSE is not recommended for use as a screening or diagnostic tool for emergent attention deficit (AD) (for example: MCI) [47]. In contrast, Montreal Cognitive Assessment (MoCA) is a brief cognitive screening tool with high sensitivity and specificity for detecting MCI, as currently conceptualized in patients performing in the normal range on the MMSE [48]. The time required for carrying out MoCA is approximately the same as for MMSE. Although none of the past studies on POCD have utilized MoCA, physicians should consider using MoCA rather than MMSE for detecting MCI preoperatively. Another promising tool is the Mini-Cog test [49]. Although this is not specifically for POCD, the American College of Surgeons National Surgical Quality Improvement Program and the American Geriatrics Society have published guidelines for optimal preoperative assessment of geriatric surgical patients [50]. The guidelines recommend obtaining a detailed history and performing a cognitive assessment, such as the Mini-Cog test, for any patient without a known history of cognitive impairment or dementia [50]. The advantages of the Mini-Cog test are its simplicity and shorter time (3–5 min) to perform the test than MMSE and MoCA. However, due to the costs involved in administering these tests, they cannot be performed in all patients. Consequently, it is very important to identify risk factors of POCD so that we can determine patients in whom the preventive measures will be effective.

6.7 Conclusion

The likely increase in the elderly population in future will also probably increase the future incidence rate of POCD. Therefore, anesthesiologists and surgeons should be aware of the possibility of POCD. Moreover, it is also important to understand the clinical status of POCD and identify patients at a high risk of developing this condition. Since efforts in this field are still in their infancy, we anticipate future progress in establishment of the tools for the screening, prevention, and treatment of POCD.

Acknowledgement Funding for this chapter was obtained from the Japan Society for the Promotion of Science, Grant-in-Aid for Scientific Research, 15K10533.

References

1. Shoair OA, Grasso Ii MP, Lahaye LA, Daniel R, Biddle CJ, Slattum PW (2015) Incidence and risk factors for postoperative cognitive dysfunction in older adults undergoing major noncardiac surgery: a prospective study. J Anaesthesiol Clin Pharmacol 31(1):30–36. doi:10.4103/0970-9185.150530
2. Krenk L, Rasmussen LS, Kehlet H (2010) New insights into the pathophysiology of postoperative cognitive dysfunction. Acta Anaesthesiol Scand 54(8):951–956. doi:10.1111/j.1399-6576.2010.02268.x
3. Bedford PD (1955) Adverse cerebral effects of anaesthesia on old people. Lancet 269(6884):259–263
4. Moller JT, Cluitmans P, Rasmussen LS, Houx P, Rasmussen H, Canet J, Rabbitt P, Jolles J, Larsen K, Hanning CD, Langeron O, Johnson T, Lauven PM, Kristensen PA, Biedler A, van Beem H, Fraidakis O, Silverstein JH, Beneken JEW, Gravenstein JS (1998) Long-term postoperative cognitive dysfunction in the elderly: ISPOCD1 study. Lancet 351(9106):857–861. doi:10.1016/s0140-6736(97)07382-0
5. Monk TG, Weldon BC, Garvan CW, Dede DE, van der Aa MT, Heilman KM, Gravenstein JS (2008) Predictors of cognitive dysfunction after major noncardiac surgery. Anesthesiology 108(1):18–30. doi:10.1097/01.anes.0000296071.19434.1e
6. Hudetz JA, Patterson KM, Amole O, Riley AV, Pagel PS (2011) Postoperative cognitive dysfunction after noncardiac surgery: effects of metabolic syndrome. J Anesth 25(3):337–344. doi:10.1007/s00540-011-1137-0
7. Chen MH, Liao Y, Rong PF, Hu R, Lin GX, Ouyang W (2013) Hippocampal volume reduction in elderly patients at risk for postoperative cognitive dysfunction. J Anesth 27(4):487–492. doi:10.1007/s00540-012-1548-6

8. Krenk L, Kehlet H, Baek Hansen T, Solgaard S, Soballe K, Rasmussen LS (2014) Cognitive dysfunction after fast-track hip and knee replacement. Anesth Analg 118(5):1034–1040. doi:10.1213/ane.0000000000000194
9. Steinmetz J, Christensen KB, Lund T, Lohse N, Rasmussen LS (2009) Long-term consequences of postoperative cognitive dysfunction. Anesthesiology 110(3):548–555. doi:10.1097/ALN.0b013e318195b569
10. Williams-Russo P, Sharrock NE, Mattis S, Szatrowski TP, Charlson ME (1995) Cognitive effects after epidural vs general anesthesia in older adults. A randomized trial. JAMA 274(1):44–50
11. Iohom G, Szarvas S, Larney V, O'Brien J, Buckley E, Butler M, Shorten G (2004) Perioperative plasma concentrations of stable nitric oxide products are predictive of cognitive dysfunction after laparoscopic cholecystectomy. Anesth Analg 99(4):1245–1252 . doi:10.1213/01.ane.0000132971.00206.4atable of contents
12. Ancelin ML, de Roquefeuil G, Ledesert B, Bonnel F, Cheminal JC, Ritchie K (2001) Exposure to anaesthetic agents, cognitive functioning and depressive symptomatology in the elderly. Br J Psychiatry 178:360–366
13. Moller JT (1997) Cerebral dysfunction after anaesthesia. Acta Anaesthesiol Scand Suppl 110:13–16
14. Hovens IB, Schoemaker RG, van der Zee EA, Heineman E, Izaks GJ, van Leeuwen BL (2012) Thinking through postoperative cognitive dysfunction: how to bridge the gap between clinical and pre-clinical perspectives. Brain Behav Immun 26(7):1169–1179. doi:10.1016/j.bbi.2012.06.004
15. Rasmussen LS (2006) Postoperative cognitive dysfunction: incidence and prevention. Best Pract Res Clin Anaesthesiol 20(2):315–330
16. Dijkstra JB, Houx PJ, Jolles J (1999) Cognition after major surgery in the elderly: test performance and complaints. Br J Anaesth 82(6):867–874
17. Sauer AM, Kalkman C, van Dijk D (2009) Postoperative cognitive decline. J Anesth 23(2):256–259. doi:10.1007/s00540-009-0744-5
18. Saito S (2013) Studies on postoperative neurological complications, particularly cognitive dysfunction. J Anesth 27(5):647–649. doi:10.1007/s00540-013-1674-9
19. Wang W, Wang Y, Wu H, Lei L, Xu S, Shen X, Guo X, Shen R, Xia X, Liu Y, Wang F (2014) Postoperative cognitive dysfunction: current developments in mechanism and prevention. Med Sci Monit 20:1908–1912. doi:10.12659/MSM.892485
20. Price CC, Garvan CW, Monk TG (2008) Type and severity of cognitive decline in older adults after noncardiac surgery. Anesthesiology 108(1):8–17. doi:10.1097/01.anes.0000296072.02527.18
21. Debess J, Riis JO, Pedersen L, Ewertz M (2009) Cognitive function and quality of life after surgery for early breast cancer in North Jutland, Denmark. Acta Oncol 48(4):532–540. doi:10.1080/02841860802600755
22. Dijkstra JB, Jolles J (2002) Postoperative cognitive dysfunction versus complaints: a discrepancy in long-term findings. Neuropsychol Rev 12(1):1–14
23. Jones MJ, Piggott SE, Vaughan RS, Bayer AJ, Newcombe RG, Twining TC, Pathy J, Rosen M (1990) Cognitive and functional competence after anaesthesia in patients aged over 60: controlled trial of general and regional anaesthesia for elective hip or knee replacement. BMJ 300(6741):1683–1687
24. Uchino H, Nagashima F, Nishiyama R, Ishida Y, Saiki I, Yara M, Hara N (2014) Pathophysiology and mechanisms of postoperative cognitive dysfunction. Masui 63(11):1202–1210
25. Deiner S, Silverstein JH (2009) Postoperative delirium and cognitive dysfunction. Br J Anaesth 103(Suppl. 1):i41–i46. doi:10.1093/bja/aep291
26. Bilotta F, Doronzio A, Stazi E, Titi L, Zeppa IO, Cianchi A, Rosa G, Paoloni FP, Bergese S, Asouhidou I, Ioannou P, Abramowicz AE, Spinelli A, Delphin E, Ayrian E, Zelman V, Lumb P (2011) Early postoperative cognitive dysfunction and postoperative delirium after anaesthesia with various hypnotics: study protocol for a randomised controlled trial—the PINOCCHIO trial. Trials 12:170. doi:10.1186/1745-6215-12-170

27. Brauer C, Morrison RS, Silberzweig SB, Siu AL (2000) The cause of delirium in patients with hip fracture. Arch Intern Med 160(12):1856–1860
28. van Harten AE, Scheeren TW, Absalom AR (2012) A review of postoperative cognitive dysfunction and neuroinflammation associated with cardiac surgery and anaesthesia. Anaesthesia 67(3):280–293. doi:10.1111/j.1365-2044.2011.07008.x
29. Riedel B, Browne K, Silbert B (2014) Cerebral protection: inflammation, endothelial dysfunction, and postoperative cognitive dysfunction. Curr Opin Anaesthesiol 27(1):89–97. doi:10.1097/aco.0000000000000032
30. Tang JX, Baranov D, Hammond M, Shaw LM, Eckenhoff MF, Eckenhoff RG (2011) Human Alzheimer and inflammation biomarkers after anesthesia and surgery. Anesthesiology 115(4):727–732. doi:10.1097/ALN.0b013e31822e9306
31. Buvanendran A, Kroin JS, Berger RA, Hallab NJ, Saha C, Negrescu C, Moric M, Caicedo MS, Tuman KJ (2006) Upregulation of prostaglandin E2 and interleukins in the central nervous system and peripheral tissue during and after surgery in humans. Anesthesiology 104(3):403–410
32. Cibelli M, Fidalgo AR, Terrando N, Ma D, Monaco C, Feldmann M, Takata M, Lever IJ, Nanchahal J, Fanselow MS, Maze M (2010) Role of interleukin-1beta in postoperative cognitive dysfunction. Ann Neurol 68(3):360–368. doi:10.1002/ana.22082
33. Wan Y, Xu J, Ma D, Zeng Y, Cibelli M, Maze M (2007) Postoperative impairment of cognitive function in rats: a possible role for cytokine-mediated inflammation in the hippocampus. Anesthesiology 106(3):436–443
34. Jin WJ, Feng SW, Feng Z, Lu SM, Qi T, Qian YN (2014) Minocycline improves postoperative cognitive impairment in aged mice by inhibiting astrocytic activation. Neuroreport 25(1):1–6. doi:10.1097/wnr.0000000000000082
35. Wang Y, He H, Li D, Zhu W, Duan K, Le Y, Liao Y, Ou Y (2013) The role of the TLR4 signaling pathway in cognitive deficits following surgery in aged rats. Mol Med Rep 7(4):1137–1142. doi:10.3892/mmr.2013.1322
36. Yirmiya R, Goshen I (2011) Immune modulation of learning, memory, neural plasticity and neurogenesis. Brain Behav Immun 25(2):181–213. doi:10.1016/j.bbi.2010.10.015
37. Terrando N, Rei Fidalgo A, Vizcaychipi M, Cibelli M, Ma D, Monaco C, Feldmann M, Maze M (2010) The impact of IL-1 modulation on the development of lipopolysaccharide-induced cognitive dysfunction. Crit Care 14(3):R88. doi:10.1186/cc9019
38. Rosczyk HA, Sparkman NL, Johnson RW (2008) Neuroinflammation and cognitive function in aged mice following minor surgery. Exp Gerontol 43(9):840–846. doi:10.1016/j.exger.2008.06.004
39. Bekker A, Lee C, de Santi S, Pirraglia E, Zaslavsky A, Farber S, Haile M, de Leon MJ (2010) Does mild cognitive impairment increase the risk of developing postoperative cognitive dysfunction? Am J Surg 199(6):782–788. doi:10.1016/j.amjsurg.2009.07.042
40. Zhu SH, Ji MH, Gao DP, Li WY, Yang JJ (2014) Association between perioperative blood transfusion and early postoperative cognitive dysfunction in aged patients following total hip replacement surgery. Ups J Med Sci 119(3):262–267. doi:10.3109/03009734.2013.873502
41. Wada-Isoe K, Uemura Y, Nakashita S, Yamawaki M, Tanaka K, Yamamoto M, Shimokata H, Nakashima K (2012) Prevalence of dementia and mild cognitive impairment in the Rural Island Town of Ama-cho, Japan. Dement Geriatr Cogn Dis Extra 2:190–199. doi:10.1159/000338244
42. Tachibana S, Hayase T, Osuda M, Kazuma S, Yamakage M (2015) Recovery of postoperative cognitive function in elderly patients after a long duration of desflurane anesthesia: a pilot study. J Anesth. doi:10.1007/s00540-015-1979-y
43. Tian Y, Zhao P, Li L, Guo Y, Wang C, Jiang Q (2014) Pre-emptive parecoxib and post-operative cognitive function in elderly patients. Int Psychogeriatr:1–8. doi:10.1017/s1041610214001951
44. Ji MH, Shen JC, Gao R, Liu XY, Yuan HM, Dong L, Wu J, Feng SW, Li WY, Yang JJ (2013) Early postoperative cognitive dysfunction is associated with higher cortisol levels in aged patients following hip fracture surgery. J Anesth 27(6):942–944. doi:10.1007/s00540-013-1633-5

45. Papadopoulos G, Karanikolas M, Liarmakopoulou A, Papathanakos G, Korre M, Beris A (2012) Cerebral oximetry and cognitive dysfunction in elderly patients undergoing surgery for hip fractures: a prospective observational study. Open Orthop J 6:400–405. doi:10.2174/1874325001206010400
46. Shu AH, Wang Q, Chen XB (2015) Effect of different depths of anesthesia on postoperative cognitive function in laparoscopic patients: a randomized clinical trial. Curr Med Res Opin 31(10):1883–1887. doi:10.1185/03007995.2015.1075968
47. Tierney MC, Szalai JP, Dunn E, Geslani D, McDowell I (2000) Prediction of probable Alzheimer disease in patients with symptoms suggestive of memory impairment. Value of the mini-mental state examination. Arch Fam Med 9(6):527–532
48. Nasreddine ZS, Phillips NA, Bedirian V, Charbonneau S, Whitehead V, Collin I, Cummings JL, Chertkow H (2005) The Montreal Cognitive Assessment, MoCA: a brief screening tool for mild cognitive impairment. J Am Geriatr Soc 53(4):695–699. doi:10.1111/j.1532-5415.2005.53221.x
49. Borson S, Scanlan J, Brush M, Vitaliano P, Dokmak A (2000) The mini-cog: a cognitive 'vital signs' measure for dementia screening in multi-lingual elderly. Int J Geriatr Psychiatry 15(11):1021–1027
50. Chow WB, Rosenthal RA, Merkow RP, Ko CY, Esnaola NF, American College of Surgeons National Surgical Quality Improvement Program, American Geriatrics Society (2012) Optimal preoperative assessment of the geriatric surgical patient: a best practices guideline from the American College of Surgeons National Surgical Quality Improvement Program and the American Geriatrics Society. J Am Coll Surg 215(4):453–466. doi:10.1016/j.jamcollsurg.2012.06.017

Chapter 7
Diagnosis of POD and POCD

Shigehito Sawamura

Abstract Postoperative delirium (POD) is a subtype of delirium that is often observed in elderly patients after surgery. Delirium is defined as an acute and fluctuating disturbance in both attention and awareness. For early diagnosis and treatment of POD, it is important to evaluate at-risk postoperative patients routinely using diagnostic tools, such as the Confusion Assessment Method (CAM), the Confusion Assessment Method for the ICU (CAM-ICU), or the Intensive Care Delirium Screening Checklist (ICDSC). The differential diagnosis of POD includes dementia, emergence delirium, and postoperative cognitive dysfunction (POCD). POCD is defined as a decline in postoperative cognitive functions as compared with preoperative functions that are evaluated by a battery of neuropsychological tests, which should be performed by trained examiners. However, there is, as yet, no consensus concerning the selection of tests, timing of postoperative testing, and diagnostic definition of decline in test scores. It is important to recognize the risk factors of both POD and POCD for prevention and early treatment of these postoperative complications that can lead to poor outcomes.

Keywords Delirium • Postoperative delirium • Postoperative cognitive dysfunction • CAM • CAM-ICU

7.1 Postoperative Delirium (POD)

POD is a subtype of delirium that is frequently observed in elderly patients after surgery. Understanding the definition and diagnosis of delirium per se is essential for the diagnosis of POD. In addition to both anesthesia and surgery,

---

S. Sawamura, M.D., Ph.D. (✉)
Department of Anesthesia, Teikyo University School of Medicine,
2-11-1 Kaga, Itabashi-ku, Tokyo 173-8605, Japan
e-mail: sawamura@med.teikyo-u.ac.jp

Y. Morimoto (ed.), *Anesthesia and Neurotoxicity*,
DOI 10.1007/978-4-431-55624-4_7

delirium is caused by many factors, including medical condition, substance intoxications/withdrawal, medications, and multiple known or unknown etiologies.

7.1.1 Definition of Delirium

Delirium is classified as one type of neurocognitive disorder in Diagnostic and Statistical Manual of Mental Disorders, Fifth Edition (DSM-5) [1], a gold standard for the diagnosis of delirium. Delirium is defined in DSM-5 as an acute and fluctuating disturbance in attention (i.e., reduced ability to direct, focus, sustain, and shift attention) and in awareness (reduced orientation to the environment). Additionally, it is accompanied with cognitive disturbances, such as memory deficit or disorientation. Moreover, the disturbance is not better explained by a preexisting, established, or evolving neurocognitive disorder (see Appendix 1 for details).

7.1.2 Diagnosis of Delirium

The clinical features often observed in delirium are shown in Table 7.1. These include an acutely changing and fluctuating level of arousal, abrupt disturbance in attention and in cognitive function, changing emotions (e.g., easy irritability,

Table 7.1 Clinical features of delirium

Acute onset and fluctuating course of the following symptoms:
1. Disturbance in attention and in awareness
Difficulty in tracking conversations and in following instructions
An inability to switch topics
Little activity or response to the environment
Drowsiness, decreased arousal, or increased arousal with hypervigilance
2. Disturbance in cognition
Memory problems, disorientation (time and place)
Difficulty in concentrating
Difficulty in speaking, recalling, reading, or writing words
Trouble in understanding speech
3. Emotional and behavioral changes
Disorganized thinking, hallucinations, paranoia
Restlessness, agitation, irritability, anxiety, depression
Sleep disturbance, reversal of the sleep/wake cycle
Slowed or decreased movement
Difficulties in maintaining postures

tearfulness), paranoid thoughts, delusions or hallucinations, decreased movement or restlessness, and sleep disturbance [2].

The diagnosis of delirium requires obtaining a current medical history, review of medical records, and laboratory and radiologic findings, and is established by several diagnostic tools. The most widely used diagnostic tools for delirium are the Confusion Assessment Method (CAM) [3] and the Confusion Assessment Method for the Intensive Care Unit (CAM-ICU) [4, 5]. The CAM-ICU is modified from the CAM for ICU patients who cannot speak due to tracheal intubation. The diagnostic criteria for delirium are shown in Appendix 2 [5]. Briefly, delirium is diagnosed if the patient (1) has an acute change or fluctuation in mental status, (2) is in a state of inattention, and either (3) has an altered level of consciousness or (4) has disorganized thinking. In clinical practice, the level of consciousness is first assessed using either the Richmond Agitation-Sedation Scale (RASS, Appendix 3) [6] or other validated sedation scales. If the patient is not in a coma or stupor (e.g., RASS −3 to +4), the evaluation proceeds to the second step, the CAM (-ICU). The diagnostic procedures of the CAM-ICU are clearly shown in an example of a CAM-ICU flow sheet (Appendix 4) [7].

The Intensive Care Delirium Screening Checklist (ICDSC) is another widely used diagnostic tool for delirium [8]. A score of 0 or 1 is given to each of the eight questions concerning (1) altered level of consciousness; (2) inattention; (3) disorientation; (4) hallucination, delusion, or psychosis; (5) psychomotor agitation or lethargy; (6) inappropriate speech or mood; (7) sleep/wake cycle disturbance; and (8) symptom fluctuation. Delirium is diagnosed if the total score is four points or more (Appendix 5). The ICDSC can easily be used by both clinicians and nurses but its relatively low specificity (64%) may lead to false positives [8].

The use of either the CAM (-ICU) or the ICDSC enables ICU nurses and physicians to diagnose delirium easily and as accurately as experts in psychiatric evaluation [5], although baseline dementia, psychosis, and anxiety/depressive disorder can sometimes make diagnosis difficult.

There are three types of delirium, including hyperactive (1.6%), hypoactive (43.5%), and mixed types (54.9%) [9]. It should be noted that the purely hyperactive type is very infrequent. The hypoactive delirium subtype is reportedly associated with the poorest outcomes.

Delirium is easily overlooked by intensive care physicians and ICU nurses unless some screening tools are used (sensitivity is 28% and 35% for physicians and nurses, respectively) [10]. Although the CAM and the CAM-ICU are validated instruments for diagnosis of delirium [11], we cannot evaluate delirium severity by these tools. Moreover, both tests have lower sensitivity when compared with their specificity [11], potentially leading to false negatives and underestimation of the incidence of the condition. We should not therefore rely solely on these screening tools, but make clinical judgments based on the DSM-5 or on other criteria for delirium.

7.1.3 Diagnosis of POD

Patients with POD usually wake up from the anesthesia initially with no problems but become delirious after a lucid interval, usually 1–3 days after surgery. These patients generally have an initial complete recovery unlike other forms of delirium. The diagnosis of POD is established when either organic or identifiable causes of delirium other than surgery are excluded.

As POD is reportedly associated with increased morbidity, prolonged hospital stay, loss of functional independence, and institutionalization, it is important to identify patients with POD and to initiate appropriate treatment as early as possible [2]. Routine (daily or during every nursing shift) assessment of postoperative patients with high POD risks using screening tools, such as the CAM-ICU, would help to diagnose and to initiate treatment of POD patients. It is recommended that health care professionals caring for postsurgical patients be trained to recognize and to document the signs and symptoms of POD, including the hypoactive type [2].

7.1.4 Differential Diagnosis for POD

Clinically, POD should be differentiated from dementia, emergence delirium, and postoperative cognitive dysfunction (POCD).

Dementia is characterized by chronic and steadily progressive disturbance in cognitive functions, while full consciousness is usually present until the last stages. These features are in contrast to the acute and fluctuating nature of POD, which is usually accompanied by an altered level of consciousness. Moreover, in contrast to POD, dementia is rarely reversible. However, dementia and POD often overlap in clinical cases.

Emergence delirium is described as a state of confusion and agitation usually lasting for 15–30 min immediately after general anesthesia. It is predominantly observed in pediatric patients under the age of 5, although young adults (<40 years) and older patients (>64 years) are also vulnerable [12].

POD should also be distinguished from postoperative cognitive dysfunction (POCD) [13], although they often overlap in clinical situations. POCD is defined by a postoperative decline in cognitive functions and, therefore, both pre- and postoperative cognitive tests are essential for the diagnosis of POCD. In contrast to POD, POCD is not necessarily accompanied by either acute or fluctuating changes in mental status. Table 7.2 summarizes the difference between POD and POCD.

7.1.5 Risk Factors for POD

An understanding of the risk factors of POD would help to foresee and to diagnose the occurrence of POD. Preoperative identification of risk factors for POD and management of the underlying risk factors are the first steps for the prevention and

Table 7.2 Differences between POD and POCD

	POD	POCD
Pathophysiology	Disturbance in attention and in awareness	Decline in cognitive functions
Diagnostic tools	CAM, CAM-ICU, ICDSC, etc.	Battery of neurocognitive tests
Onset/course	Acute/fluctuating	Subtle/stable
Symptoms	Relatively clear (unclear in hypoactive cases)	Unclear, often clarified only by cognitive tests
Periods	Days to weeks, resolves completely	Weeks to months (sometimes lasting forever)
Risk factors	Age, severe illness, baseline dementia, infection, dehydration, hearing or visual loss, pain, restraint	Age, baseline dementia, inflammation
Treatment	Possible (pharmacological and nonpharmacological)	Unknown at present
Prevention	Possible by multimodal interventions	Unknown at present

Table 7.3 Risk factors for POD

Age >65
Preoperative cognitive impairment
Severe illness
Previous history of delirium
Hearing or vision impairment
Presence of infection
Inadequately controlled pain
Immobilization or limited mobility
Depression, alcohol abuse, sleep disturbance
Polypharmacy and use of psychotropic medications (benzodiazepines, anticholinergics, antihistamines, antipsychotics)
Renal insufficiency
Anemia, poor nutrition, electrolyte and fluid abnormalities
Presence of urinary catheter
Vascular or aortic procedures
Current hip fracture
ICU admission

treatment of POD. Risk factors include older age, baseline cognitive impairment, severe illness, hearing or vision impairment, infection, alcohol abuse, pain, and sleep disturbances (Table 7.3) [2, 14].

7.2 Postoperative Cognitive Dysfunction (POCD)

Elderly patients often experience decline in cognitive functions for weeks to months after surgery. POCD refers to deterioration in cognitive functions temporally associated with surgery. Cognitive functions are evaluated using a battery of neuropsychological tests, although patient complaints or observations by family members sometimes provide useful information.

Initially, attention was paid to POCD after cardiac surgery. However, it is now known that POCD can occur not only after on-pump cardiac surgery, but also following off-pump cardiac surgery or even following noncardiac surgery [15]. Diagnosis of POCD is important because it is known to be associated with a diminished quality of life and with increased mortality after surgery [16].

7.2.1 *Symptoms of POCD*

In contrast to the acute and sometimes obvious onset of POD, POCD usually manifests itself as a subtle decline in cognitive functions, including memory, attention, concentration, perception, verbal function, learning, and social activities. Cognitive declines are often revealed only by a comparison of pre- and postoperative neuropsychological test scores. Therefore, subjective self-reported cognitive symptoms do not substitute for an objective cognitive evaluation.

7.2.2 *Diagnosis of POCD*

Although patient complaints or family observations sometimes suggest the occurrence of POCD, the diagnosis of POCD is established only through comparison of pre- and postoperative scores in a battery of neuropsychological tests. Therefore, to diagnose POCD correctly, patients need to have been tested using preoperative cognitive examinations, which is not usually the case in clinical practice. At present, there is no established consensus concerning the optimum selection of neuropsychological tests, suitable timing of postoperative examinations, or criteria for defining the “decline” in test scores.

7.2.3 *Neuropsychological Tests*

As multiple locations of the brain can be influenced to various extents in POCD, it is important to select an efficient combination of neuropsychological tests to evaluate several cognitive domains and to diagnose POCD correctly.

Although, as yet, there is no standardized neurocognitive test batteries routinely used for the diagnosis of POCD, a consensus meeting in 1995 advocated four core tests as detailed below (Sects. 7.2.3.1–7.2.3.3) [17].

7.2.3.1 Rey Auditory Verbal Learning Test for Verbal Memory

The examiner reads aloud a list of 15 words, and then the participant is asked to repeat all the words he or she can remember in any order. The procedure is carried out five times. Then a second list of 15 words is presented and the participant attempts to recall them (only once for this time). Immediately following this, the participant is asked to remember as many words as possible from the first list.

7.2.3.2 Trail-Making A and Trail-Making B for Attention and Concentration

These tests consist of 25 circled numbers or letters distributed over a sheet of paper (1 to 25 for Test A, 1 to 13 and A to L for Test B). The participant is asked to draw lines to connect circles in ascending order as quickly as possible (1-2-3-4- for Test A, 1-A-2-B-3-C- for Test B).

7.2.3.3 Grooved Pegboard Test for Motor Skills

This test involves a pegboard with 25 holes with randomly positioned slots and pegs with a key along one side. The participant is asked to pick up a peg, rotate it, and insert it to match the hole with one hand. The time to insert all of the 25 pegs correctly into the holes is measured.

7.2.3.4 Other Tests

Other cognitive tests often used to diagnose POCD include the Stroop test (the word red is printed in blue ink, for example; you are asked to name the color of the ink instead of the word itself), the digit span test for short-term memory (how many digits of numbers the subject can remember), and the paper and pencil memory test for sensorimotor and recall speed. The Mini-Mental Status Examination (MMSE) takes only 5 min and is considered to be suitable for preoperative identification of subclinical dementia. However, the MMSE is fundamentally a screening tool and may not be sensitive enough to detect a subtle postoperative decline in cognitive function. Furthermore, the MMSE is not suitable for quantitative evaluation of POCD because there is a learning effect caused by repeated examinations.

Neurocognitive tests should be conducted by trained and qualified examiners to reduce variance in scores that cannot be ascribed to the subjects' ability alone. Moreover, anxiety and depression should also be assessed because these conditions are known to affect cognitive performance. Lastly, it should be noted that many of the neuropsychological tests are not designed to detect the subtle cognitive impairment seen in surgical patients.

7.2.4 Evaluation of the Neuropsychological Test Scores

Most previous studies on POCD have defined "positive decline" in cognitive tests as "more than a 20% decrease in test scores" or "decrease of more than once or twice the standard deviation of control patients' scores" [18]. Recent studies calculate a Z-score of a patient's postoperative score change from the mean and standard deviation of score changes in a control group and assume a $Z < -1.96$ (or -2) as "positive decline." Making a matched control group can thus be helpful for defining the "decline" in neuropsychological tests. It removes the normal variations of test scores, learning effects induced by repeated testing, and effects of aging in the same patients. However, it should be noted that selected controls do not always match the surgical populations well.

In many studies, POCD has been defined as a positive decline in more than two of the neuropsychological tests performed. Although it is clear that employing a single neuropsychological test is insufficient to diagnose POCD, increasing the number of tests can also cause a problem. When POCD was defined as "decline in scores in more than two of the neuropsychological tests performed," increasing the total number of tests from two to seven increased the incidence of POCD from 3 to 41% even in the control group [19]. Increasing the number of tests can thus increase the possibility of "false positives," and the incidence of POCD can thus be overestimated [20].

7.2.5 Timing of Examinations

The decline in cognitive function is usually most prominent in the immediate postoperative period and then recovers gradually. It lasts for weeks or months and sometimes forever. The incidence of POCD is reportedly 26–41% and 10–13% at 1 week and at 3 months after surgery, respectively, in patients over age 60 [15, 21]. Therefore, to observe the time course of POCD, neuropsychological tests should be performed at least once during the stable period, that is, more than 3 months after the surgery. There is no rigid consensus concerning the optimum time points of examinations. However, it may be difficult to diagnose early POCD (a few days postoperatively), because the patient can be in delirium or still under the influence of anesthetics, analgesics, pain, or fatigue.

Table 7.4 Risk factors for POCD

Risk factors
Advanced age
Preoperative mild cognitive impairment
Lower educational level
Previous stroke with no residual damage
Alcohol abuse
Extensive surgical procedure
Preoperative cerebral, cardiac, or vascular disease
Use of multiple medications
Delirium
Depression

7.2.6 Risk Factors of POCD

Although the etiology to POCD is still unknown, recognizing the risk factors of POCD would greatly help to foresee, detect, or sometimes prevent the occurrence of POCD. The incidence of POCD is independent of the type of either surgery or anesthesia [22]. The risk factors for POCD reported in previous studies [21] are shown in Table 7.4. Of these risk factors, patient age has been the most consistently mentioned.

Appendix 1. Definition of Delirium by DSM-5 [1]

A. Disturbance in attention (i.e., reduced ability to direct, focus, sustain, and shift attention) and awareness (reduced orientation to the environment).
B. The disturbance develops over a short period of time (usually hours to a few days), represents an acute change from baseline attention and awareness, and tends to fluctuate in severity during the course of a day.
C. An additional disturbance in cognition (e.g., memory deficit, disorientation, language, visuospatial ability, or perception).
D. The disturbances in Criteria A and C are not better explained by a preexisting, established, or evolving neurocognitive disorder and do not occur in the context of a severely reduced level of arousal such as coma.
E. There is evidence from the history, physical examination, or laboratory findings that the disturbance is a direct physiological consequence of another medical condition, substance intoxication or withdrawal (i.e., due to a drug of abuse or to a medication), or exposure to a toxin, or is due to multiple etiologies.

Appendix 2. The Confusion Assessment Method for the Intensive Care Unit (CAM-ICU) [5] (Reprinted with permission)

Delirium is diagnosed when both Features 1 and 2 are positive, along with either Feature 3 or Feature 4.

Feature 1.

Acute Onset of Mental Status Changes or Fluctuating Course.

Is there evidence of an acute change in mental status from the baseline?

Did the (abnormal) behavior fluctuate during the past 24 h, that is, tend to come and go or increase and decrease in severity?

Sources of information: Serial Glasgow Coma Scale or sedation score ratings over 24 h as well as readily available input from the patient's bedside critical care nurse or family.

Feature 2.

Inattention.

Did the patient have difficulty focusing attention?

Is there a reduced ability to maintain and shift attention?

Sources of information: Attention screening examinations by using either picture recognition or Vigilance A random letter test (see Methods and Appendix 2 for description of Attention Screening Examinations). Neither of these tests requires verbal response, and thus they are ideally suited for mechanically ventilated patients.

Feature 3.

Disorganized Thinking.

Was the patient's thinking disorganized or incoherent, such as rambling or irrelevant conversation, unclear or illogical flow of ideas, or unpredictable switching from subject to subject?

Was the patient able to follow questions and commands throughout the assessment?

1. "Are you having any unclear thinking?"
2. "Hold up this many fingers." (examiner holds two fingers in front of the patient)
3. "Now, do the same thing with the other hand." (not repeating the number of fingers)

Feature 4.

Altered level of consciousness.

Any level of consciousness other than "alert."

Alert—normal, spontaneously fully aware of environment and interacts appropriately.

Vigilant—hyperalert.

Lethargic—drowsy but easily aroused, unaware of some elements in the environment, or not spontaneously interacting appropriately with the interviewer; becomes fully aware and appropriately interactive when prodded minimally.

Stupor—difficult to arouse, unaware of some or all elements in the environment, or not spontaneously interacting with the interviewer; becomes incompletely aware and inappropriately interactive when prodded strongly.

Coma—unarousable, unaware of all elements in the environment, with no spontaneous interaction or awareness of the interviewer, so that the interview is difficult or impossible even with maximal prodding.

Appendix 3. Richmond Agitation Sedation Scale (RASS) [6]

Score	Term	Description
+4	Combative	Overtly combative or violent; immediate danger to staff
+3	Very agitation	Pulls on or removes tube(s) or catheter(s) or has aggressive behavior toward staff
+2	Agitated	Frequent nonpurposeful movement or patient–ventilator dyssynchrony
+1	Restless	Anxious or apprehensive but movements not aggressive or vigorous
0	Alert and calm	
−1	Drowsy	Not fully alert, but has sustained (more than 10 s) awakening, with eye contact, to voice
−2	Light sedation	Briefly (less than 10 s) awakens with eye contact to voice
−3	Moderate sedation	Any movement (but no eye contact) to voice
−4	Deep sedation	No response to voice, but any movement to physical stimulation
−5	Unarousable	No response to voice or physical stimulation

Procedure
1. Observe patient. Is patient alert and calm (score 0)?
Does patient have behavior that is consistent with restlessness or agitation (score +1 to +4 using the criteria listed above, under DESCRIPTION)?
2. If patient is not alert, in a loud speaking voice state patient' s name and direct patient to open eyes and look at speaker. Repeat once if necessary. Can prompt patient to continue looking at speaker.
Patient has eye opening and eye contact, which is sustained for more than 10 s (score −1).
Patient has eye opening and eye contact, but this is not sustained for 10 s (score −2).
Patient has any movement in response to voice, excluding eye contact (score −3).
3. If patient does not respond to voice, physically stimulate patient by shaking shoulder and then rubbing sternum if there is no response to shaking shoulder.
Patient has any movement to physical stimulation (score −4).
Patient has no response to voice or physical stimulation (score −5).

Appendix 4. An Example of CAM-ICU Flow Sheet [7] (Reprinted with permission)

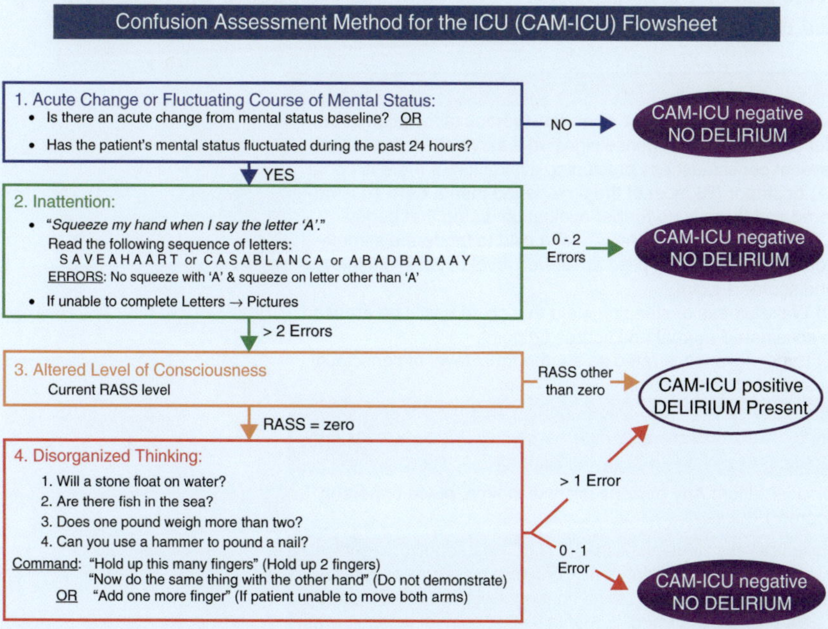

Appendix 5. Intensive Care Delirium Screening Checklist (ICDSC) [8] (With permission of Springer)

A score of 0 or 1 is given to each of the eight questions above and delirium is diagnosed if the total score is four points or more.

1. Altered level of consciousness:
   A) No response or B) the need for vigorous stimulation in order to obtain any response signified a serve alteration in the level of consciousness precluding evaluation. If there is coma (A) or stupor (B) most of the time period then a dash (-) is entered and there is no further evaluation during that period.
   C) Drowsiness or requirement of a mild to moderate stimulation for a response implies an altered level of consciousness and scores 1 point.
   D) Wakefulness or sleeping state that could easily be aroused is considered normal and scores no point.
   E) Hypervigilance is rated as an abnormal level of consciousness and scored 1 point.
2. Inattention: Difficulty in following a conversation or instrutions. Easily distracted by external stimuli. Difficulty in shifting focuses. Any of these scores 1 point.
3. Disorientation: Any obvious mistake in time, place or person scores 1 point.
4. Hallucination, delusion or psychosis: The unequivocal clinical manifestation of hallucination or of behavior probably due to hallucination (e.g., trying to catch a non-existent object) or delusion. Gross impairment in reality testing. Any of these scores 1 point.
5. Psychomotor agitation or retardation: Hyperactivity requiring the use of additional sedative drugs or restraints in order to control potential danger to oneself or others (e.g., pulling out iv lines, hitting staff). Hypoactivity or clinically noticeable psychomotor slowing. Any of these scores 1 point.
6. Inappropriate speech or mood: Inappropriate, disorganized or incoherent speech. Inappropriate display of emotion related to events or situation. Any of these scores 1 point.
7. Sleep/wake cycle disturbance: Sleeping less than 4 h or waking frequently at night (do not consider wakefulness initiated by medical staff or loud environment). Sleeping during most of the day. Any of these scores 1 point.
8. Symptom fluctuation: Fluctuation of the manifestation of any item or symptom over 24 h (e.g., from one shift to another) scores 1 point.

References

1. American Psychiatric Association (2013) Diagnostic and statistical manual of mental disorders, 5th edn. DSM–5. American Psychiatric Association Publishing, Arlington, VA
2. American Geriatrics Society Expert Panel on Postoperative Delirium in Older Adults (2015) Postoperative delirium in older adults: best practice statement from the American geriatrics society. J Am Coll Surg 220(2):136–148.e1. doi:10.1016/j.jamcollsurg.2014.10.019
3. Inouye SK, van Dyck CH, Alessi CA et al (1990) Clarifying confusion: the confusion assessment method. A new method for detection of delirium. Ann Intern Med 113(12):941–948
4. Ely EW, Inouye SK, Bernard GR et al (2001) Delirium in mechanically ventilated patients: validity and reliability of the confusion assessment method for the intensive care unit (CAM-ICU). JAMA 286(21):2703–2710. doi:10.1001/jama.286.21.2703
5. Ely EW, Margolin R, Francis J et al (2001) Evaluation of delirium in critically ill patients: Validation of the confusion assessment method for the intensive care unit (CAM-ICU). Crit Care Med 29(7):1370–1379
6. Sessler CN, Gosnell MS, Grap MJ et al (2002) The Richmond agitation-sedation scale: validity and reliability in adult intensive care unit patients. Am J Respir Crit Care Med 166(10):1338–1344. doi:10.1164/rrcm.2107138
7. Ely EW, Vanderbilt University (2014) Confusion assessment method for the ICU (CAM-ICU). The complete training manual. Revised edition: March 2014. Available via http://www.icudelirium.org/docs/CAM_ICU_flowsheet.pdf. Accessed 26 Nov 2015
8. Bergeron N, Dubois MJ, Dumont M et al (2001) Intensive care delirium screening checklist: evaluation of a new screening tool. Intensive Care Med 27(5):859–864. doi:10.1007/s001340100909
9. Peterson JF, Pun BT, Dittus RS et al (2006) Delirium and its motoric subtypes: a study of 614 critically ill patients. J Am Geriatr Soc 54(3):479–484. doi:10.1111/j.1532-5415.2005.00621.x
10. Spronk PE, Riekerk B, Hofhuis J et al (2009) Occurrence of delirium is severely underestimated in the ICU during daily care. Intensive Care Med 35(7):1276–1280. doi:10.1007/s00134-009-1466-8
11. Shi Q, Warren L, Saposnik G et al (2013) Confusion assessment method: a systematic review and meta-analysis of diagnostic accuracy. Neuropsychiatr Dis Treat 9:1359–1370. doi:10.2147/NDT.S49520
12. Munk L, Andersen LP, Gögenur I (2013) Emergence delirium. J Perioper Pract 23(11): 251–254
13. Krenk L, Rasmussen LS (2011) Postoperative delirium and postoperative cognitive dysfunction in the elderly—what are the differences? Minerva Anestesiol 77(7):742–749
14. Dasgupta M, Dumbrell AC (2006) Preoperative risk assessment for delirium after noncardiac surgery: a systematic review. J Am Geriatr Soc 54(10):1578–1589. doi:10.1111/j1532-5415.2006.00893.x
15. Moller JT, Cluitmans P, Rasmussen LS et al (1998) Long-term postoperative cognitive dysfunction in the elderly ISPOCD1 study. ISPOCD investigators. International study of postoperative cognitive dysfunction. Lancet 351(9106):857–861
16. Steinmetz J, Christensen KB, Lund T et al (2009) Long-term consequences of postoperative cognitive dysfunction. Anesthesiology 110(3):548–555. doi:10.1097/ALN.0b013e318195b569
17. Murkin JM, Newman SP, Stump DA et al (1995) Statement of consensus on assessment of neurobehavioral outcomes after cardiac surgery. Ann Thorac Surg 59(5):1289–1295
18. Rudolph JL, Schreiber KA, Culley DJ et al (2010) Measurement of post-operative cognitive dysfunction after cardiac surgery: a systematic review. Acta Anaesthesiol Scand 54(6):663–677. doi:10.1111/j.1399-6576.2010.02236.x
19. Lewis MS, Maruff P, Silbert BS et al (2006) Detection of postoperative cognitive decline after coronary artery bypass graft surgery is affected by the number of neuropsychological tests in the assessment battery. Ann Thorac Surg 81(6):2097–2104. doi:10.1016/j.athoracsur.2006.01.044

20. Selnes OA, Gottesman RF, Grega MA et al (2012) Cognitive and neurologic outcomes after coronary-artery bypass surgery. N Engl J Med 366(3):250–257. doi:10.1056/NEJMra1100109
21. Monk TG, Weldon BC, Garvan CW et al (2008) Predictors of cognitive dysfunction after major noncardiac surgery. Anesthesiology 108(1):18–30
22. Evered L, Scott DA, Silbert B et al (2011) Postoperative cognitive dysfunction is independent of type of surgery and anesthetic. Anesth Analg 112(5):1179–1185. doi:10.1213/ANE.0b013e318215217e

Chapter 8
Prevention and Treatment of Postoperative Delirium and Postoperative Cognitive Dysfunction

Mitsuru Ida and Masahiko Kawaguchi

Abstract Postoperative delirium (POD) is a common complication of surgery and an acute and fluctuating neurological disorder that is characterized by disturbances of consciousness, attention, and perception. Postoperative cognitive dysfunction (POCD) is a subtle transient cognitive decline that occurs for weeks or months after surgery. POCD may influence isolated cognition domains, such as verbal memory, visual memory, attention, and concentration, and is not necessarily accompanied by a change in consciousness. Although POD is a transient and curable clinical condition, it may encompass POCD and increase postoperative mortality. Saczynski et al. demonstrated that patients with POD had more severe POCD at 1 week and 1 year after surgery and that the longer the POD continued, the worse the cognitive dysfunction. Prevention and treatment of POD may prevent POCD. POCD influences both the short-term and long-term prognosis. Patients with POCD at 1 week after surgery had greater difficulty returning to work and tended to receive social transfer payments, whereas those with POCD at 3 months after surgery were associated with increased mortality. In this chapter, we describe POD and POCD and particularly focus on their prevention and treatment.

Keywords Postoperative delirium • Postoperative cognitive dysfunction • Drug/Nondrug therapy

---

M. Ida (✉) • M. Kawaguchi
Department of Anesthesiology, Nara Medical University,
840 Shijo-cho, Kashihara, Nara 634-8522, Japan
e-mail: nwnh0131@yahoo.co.jp

Y. Morimoto (ed.), *Anesthesia and Neurotoxicity*,
DOI 10.1007/978-4-431-55624-4_8

8.1 Postoperative Delirium

8.1.1 Incidence

The total incidence of POD is 36.8%, with the incidence varying depending on the type of surgery [1]. For example, POD was reported in 16–44% patients undergoing hip fracture repair and 29–39% patients undergoing vascular surgery [2]. Delirium is classified as hyperactive or hypoactive, with hypoactive delirium being more difficult to recognize. Therefore, POD incidence may be underestimated.

8.1.2 Predictors

Table 8.1 shows the risk model of POD in noncardiac surgery [3]. Additional risk factors include emergency surgery [4], laboratory abnormalities (sodium, potassium, and glucose) [5], a history of hypertension, and higher acute physiology and chronic health evaluation II scores [6].

8.1.3 Mechanism [7]

While the mechanism underlying POD is unknown, it is thought to involve altered neurotransmission, inflammation, and chronic stress. Cholinergic and dopaminergic neurotransmitters are involved in POD. Inflammatory cytokines, such as

Table 8.1. The risk model for delirium [3]

Predisposing risk factors for delirium	Points
Delirium during previous hospitalization	5
Dementia	5
Clock drawing (displaying 10 past 11)	
Small mistakes	1
Big mistakes, unrecognizable, or no attempt	2
Age	
70–85 years	1
>85 years	2
Impaired hearing (patient is not able to hear speech)	1
Impaired vision (vision <40%)	1
Problems in activities of daily live	
Domestic help or help with meal preparation	0.5
Help with physical care	0.5
Use of heroin, methadone, or morphine	2
Daily consumption of four or more alcoholic beverages	2

Patients scoring 5 or more points were considered high risk for postoperative delirium interleukin-6 and -8 and tumor necrosis factor α, increase the permeability of the blood–brain barrier, resulting in changes in neurotransmission. Furthermore, chronic surgical stress increases cortisol release, which may have an effect on POD.

8.1.4 Anesthetics

A meta-analysis that compared the influence of general anesthesia, local anesthesia, and a combination of these on POD reported that general anesthesia did not increase the incidence of POD (OR 0.88; 95% CI, 0.51–1.51) [8]. A randomized controlled trial that compared the effects of propofol and sevoflurane on POD after laparoscopic surgery revealed that POD incidence during the first 3 days was comparable; however, the delirium rating scale, 2 and 3 days after surgery, was significantly higher after propofol than after sevoflurane anesthesia [9]. Monitoring of anesthesia via electroencephalogram was shown to decrease POD incidence [10, 11], possibly due to the use of less anesthetic; however, the exact mechanism is unknown. Some drugs used perioperatively, such as atropine, antihistamines, corticosteroids, and benzodiazepines, can precipitate delirium; therefore, their use should be minimized [12].

8.1.5 Prevention

8.1.5.1 Nondrug Therapy

Environmental change is closely associated with POD, and clinicians should pay attention to adjusting environmental factors (Table 8.2) [13]. Two reports have shown that proactive geriatric consultation can decrease POD risk. In one study [14], 126 patients who underwent hip fracture repair were randomly assigned to proactive geriatric consultation or standard treatment. Geriatric consultation involved daily patient visits with a geriatrician during hospitalization and interventions based on a structured protocol. POD incidence was lower in patients

Table 8.2. Environmental coordination to prevent postoperative delirium [13]

Keep adequate lighting during the day
Recognize the date, time, and location at least three times a day
Provide the clock and calendar
Wear hearing aids and glasses if necessary
Nursing continually
Early ambulation
Reduce noise
Meet with family
Prevent dehydration
Regulate bowel function
Give supplemental oxygen to keep saturation >95%

undergoing geriatric consultation than in controls (32% vs. 50%; $P = 0.04$) with a relative risk of 0.64 (95% CI, 0.37–0.98). The incidence of severe POD was also lower in patients undergoing geriatric consultation than in controls (12% vs. 29%; $P = 0.02$) with a relative risk of 0.4 (95% CI, 0.18–0.89). In another study [15], 199 patients with femoral neck fracture were randomly assigned to postoperative care in a specialized geriatric ward or an orthopedic ward. Patients in the geriatric ward had a lower incidence of POD (54.9% vs. 75.3%; $P = 0.003$) and a shorter POD duration (5.0 days vs. 10.2 days; $P = 0.009$).

8.1.5.2 Drug Therapy [16] (Table 8.3)

Many reports discuss the use of drugs to prevent POD.

Patients who were administered haloperidol (0.1 mg/h for 12 h) after a 0.5 mg injection had a significantly lower incidence of POD (5.3% vs. 23.2%; $P = 0.031$) [17]. However, the effectiveness of haloperidol depended on the type of surgery, and the reduction was only confirmed in patients who underwent abdominal surgery in this study. In another study, patients undergoing cardiac surgery with cardiopulmonary bypass were randomly assigned to sublingually receive either 1 mg risperidone or placebo upon regaining consciousness. The incidence of POD was lower in patients treated with risperidone than placebo (11.1% vs. 31.7%; $P = 0.009$; RR, 0.35; 95% CI, 0.16–0.77) [18]. Olanzapine and risperidone both block dopamine-2 and serotonin receptors, and their prophylactic use may be effective in preventing POD. Four hundred patients who underwent noncardiac surgery were randomly assigned to directly receive either olanzapine (5 mg) or placebo preceding and after surgery. The incidence of POD was significantly lower in the olanzapine group (14.3% vs. 40.2; $P < 0.0001$; 95% CI, 17.6–34.2) [19].

Intramuscular injection of diazepam at 8 p.m. each night followed by continuous administration of flunitrazepam and pethidine over 8 h was reported to decrease POD incidence but increase the incidence of morning lethargy [20]. Midazolam had no effect on POD [21].

Table 8.3. Summary of prevention strategies of postoperative delirium

Proactive geriatric consultation
Haloperidol injection (0.5 mg) with subsequent administration (0.1 mg/h) for 12 h
Risperidone (1 mg) sublingually when they regained consciousness
Olanzapine (5 mg) just before and after surgery
Melatonin (5 mg) at sleep time and another 5 mg 90 min prior to operation
Oral gabapentin (900 mg) administered 1–2 h before surgery
Remifentanil or fascia iliaca compartment block
Dexmedetomidine

Because of the association of Parkinson's and Alzheimer's disease with excess cholinergic activity, several studies have investigated whether cholinesterase inhibitors decrease POD risk. However, neither donepezil (5 mg) administration 14 days before and after surgery [22] nor rivastigmine (1.5 mg) administration for three consecutive days starting the evening before surgery decreased POD incidence [23].

The sleep–wake cycle is closely associated with delirium. One study focusing on the association between sleep–wake cycle disruptions and plasma melatonin revealed that melatonin administration (5 mg) at sleep time and 90 min before surgery decreased POD incidence (9.43% vs. 32.65%) and was helpful for treating patients who had developed POD [21].

The oral administration of gabapentin (900 mg) 1–2 h before surgery was reported to be safe and was associated with a significantly lower POD incidence and pain-level improvement (0% vs. 42%; $P = 0.045$) [24].

Remifentanil is reportedly associated with a lower POD incidence than fentanyl in the recovery room ($P = 0.039$) and on the first postoperative day ($P = 0.005$) [25]. Furthermore, in patients undergoing surgical hip-fracture repair, administration of a fascia iliaca compartment block before initiating surgery until delirium occurred or until the patient underwent surgery decreased POD incidence (10.8% vs. 23.8%; RR 0.45; 95% CI, 0.23–0.87) [24].

A meta-analysis revealed that dexmedetomidine administration decreased the incidence of delirium, agitation, and confusion (19% vs. 23%; $P = 0.03$; RR, 0.68; 95% CI, 0.49–0.96) [26].

8.1.6 *Treatment*

Prevention is the best approach because treatments for POD are still under investigation. A recent meta-analysis demonstrated that antipsychotics decrease the incidence of postoperative delirium [27]. Several studies have evaluated the effectiveness of drugs in treating POD; for example, quetiapine plus haloperidol resulted in faster delirium resolution [28]. However most of these studies had small cohorts and were unable to determine which drugs are preferable. Rivastigmine did not decrease delirium duration over that of haloperidol and showed evidence of increased mortality [29]. Treatment strategies are shown in Table 8.4.

Table 8.4. Summary of treatment strategies for postoperative delirium [7]

Search for and correct the causes of delirium
Intravenous or subcutaneous injection of haloperidol (2.5 mg)
Oral haloperidol (1–2 mg) every 4 h
Oral olanzapine (2.5–5 mg) daily
Oral risperidone (0.5–1 mg) daily (for elderly patients, cut dose by 25–50%)
Benzodiazepines (in case of delirium due to benzodiazepine withdrawal, alcohol withdrawal, or postseizure delirium)

8.2 Postoperative Cognitive Dysfunction

8.2.1 *Incidence*

The International Study of Post-Operative Cognitive Dysfunction 1 evaluated the incidence of POCD in 1218 patients aged ≥60 years who underwent abdominal, orthopedic, or thoracic surgery and revealed that POCD was experienced by 25.8% of these patients on postoperative day 7 and 9.9% at 3 months after surgery [30]. The incidence of POCD in these patients was significantly higher than that of healthy controls ($P < 0.0001$, $P = 0.0037$). Similarly, among 336 patients aged ≥60 years, POCD was present in 24.8% at 1 week, 10.3% at 3 months, and 10.4% at 1–2 years after surgery [31]. POCD occurs not only in elderly patients but also in middle-aged and young patients. In a study of 1064 noncardiac surgery patients aged 18–39, 40–59, and ≥60 years, POCD was found in all age groups, and the prevalence of POCD decreased with time after surgery [32].

8.2.2 *Predictors*

The risk factors of POCD are shown in Tables 8.5, 8.6, and 8.7 [30, 31] according to postoperative terms. Age was the most significant predictor of POCD in all terms. In addition to the listed factors, cognitive functions are more

Table 8.5. Risk factors related to postoperative cognitive function at 1 week after surgery [33]

Risk factor	*P*-value	Odds ratio (95% confidence interval)
Age (difference of 10 years)	0.03	1.3 (1.0–1.7)
Anesthesia time (difference of 1 h)	0.01	1.1 (1.0–1.3)
Second surgery in 1 week	0.03	2.7 (1.1–6.5)
Postoperative respiratory complication	0.05	1.6 (1.0–2.6)
Postoperative infectious complication	0.04	1.7 (1.0–2.8)
Education level (high school vs. less than high school)	0.002	0.6 (0.4–0.9)

Table 8.6. Risk factors related to postoperative cognitive function at 1 week after surgery [33]

Risk factor	*P*-value	Odds ratio (95% confidence interval)
Age (difference of 10 years)	0.0001	2.1 (1.4–2.9)
Benzodiazepines before surgery	0.03	0.4 (0.2–1.0)

Table 8.7. Risk factors related to postoperative cognitive function in 1–2 years after surgery [31]

Risk factor	*P*-value	Odds ratio (95% confidence interval)
Age (difference of 10 years)	0.002	2.58 (1.42–4.70)
Postoperative infectious complication	0.045	2.61 (1.02–6.68)
Presence of POCD at 1 week after surgery	0.006	2.84 (1.35–5.96)

POCD postoperative cognitive function

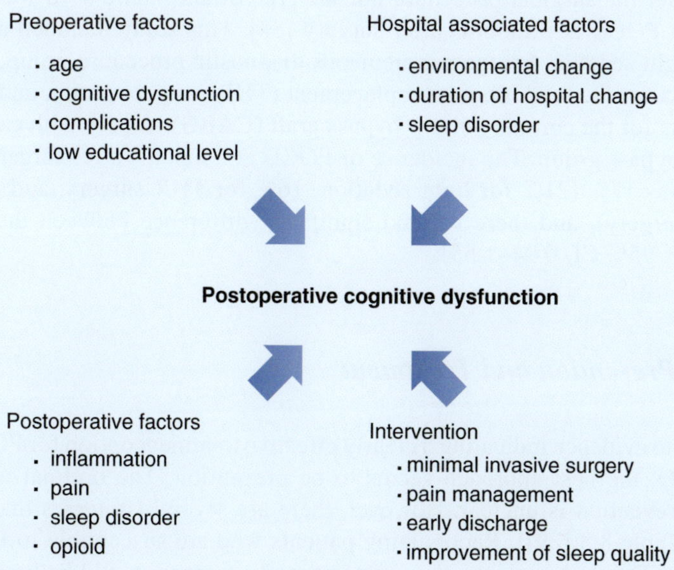

Fig. 8.1. Intraoperative factors and interventions for postoperative cognitive dysfunction [35]

profoundly impaired in patients with a history of alcohol abuse [33] or with metabolic syndrome [34].

8.2.3 Mechanism

Various factors are associated with POCD (Fig. 8.1) [35]. Inflammation plays an important role in POCD. Inflammatory cytokines induced by surgery affect not only the surgical area but also the central nervous system, disrupting the blood–brain barrier and resulting in POCD. An animal study comparing the incidence of POCD between general anesthesia alone and general anesthesia with surgery revealed that systematic inflammation caused by surgical trauma rather than the influence of general anesthesia was strongly related to POCD [36].

8.2.4 Anesthetics

In a study investigating the incidence of mental changes in epidural versus general anesthesia for total hip arthroplasty in 60 elderly patients, the author concluded that epidural anesthesia should be selected because only 7 of the 31 patients in the general anesthesia group experienced postoperative mental changes [37]. In contrast, a recent prospective observational study suggested that neither the surgical procedure nor the type of anesthetic used was associated with POCD at 3 months after surgery [38]. This study included a control group, light sedation for the percutaneous diagnostic procedure group, general anesthesia for the total hip joint replacement (THR) surgery group, and general anesthesia for the coronary artery bypass graft (CABG) surgery with cardiopulmonary bypass group. The incidence of POCD at 3 months after surgery for all groups was 17% (21% for light sedation, 16% for THR surgery, and 16% for CABG surgery), and there was no significant difference between the groups (OR 1.21; 95% CI, 0.94–1.55).

8.2.5 Prevention and Treatment

There is no evidence indicating a clearly effective treatment option for POCD. As with POD, the best approach seems to be prevention. The optimal means of POCD prevention is unclear. However, there are several strategies that reduce POCD (Table 8.8 [39]). Recognizing patients who are susceptible to POCD is important. For such patients, the use of benzodiazepines should be limited, and the preoperative fasting time should be shortened. Considering the relationship between POCD and inflammation, inhibiting inflammation may help to reduce POCD. Evidence from studies in animals [40–43] and humans [44, 45] suggests

Table 8.8. Prevention strategies for postoperative cognitive dysfunction [39]

Maintain homeostasis
Avoid benzodiazepines
Minimal invasive surgery
Short surgery time
Early discharge
Frequent explanation
Pain control
Avoid long-term fasting
Frequent visiting with family or friends

Table 8.9. Drugs expected to prevent POCD

First author [Ref]	Drug	Object	Intervention	Main result
Tian [40]	Vitamin D	Mice	Partial hepatectomy under general anesthesia	Useful in the control of inflammatory diseases
Jin [41]	Minocycline	Mice	70% partial hepatectomy	Improved postoperative memory impairment
				Inhibited astrocytic activation induced
				Downregulated TNF-a, IL-1b, and IL-6 mRNA expression levels
Zhang [42]	Amantadine	Rat	Right carotid exposure under intravenous anesthesia	Attenuated surgery-induced learning and memory impairment
Sun [44]	Dobutamine	Human	Total hip arthroplasty under epidural anesthesia	Prevented surgery-induced POCD
				Reduced anesthesia-induced TNF-α release in patient plasma
Ottens [47]	Dexamethasone (0.1 mg/kg)	Human	Cardiac surgery with cardiopulmonary bypass	Did not reduce the risk of POCD
Fang [46]	Dexamethasone (0.2 mg/kg)	Human	Microvascular decompression	Increased the incidence of POCD
Kawano [43]	Ketoprofen	Rat	Postoperative pain model	Prevented the development of surgery-associated memory deficits
Tian [45]	Parecoxib	Human	Orthopedic surgery under general anesthesia	Reduced the incidence of POCD

TNF tumor necrosis factor, *IL* interleukin, *POCD* postoperative cognitive function

several drugs that may help for preventing POCD (Table 8.9). In contrast, dexamethasone (0.2 mg/kg) may increase the incidence of POCD [46] or have no effect [47].

The surgical technique used may affect the risk of POCD. A meta-analysis demonstrated no difference in POCD incidence between off-pump CABG and on-pump CABG surgery [48]; however, the occurrence of POCD after cardiac surgeries is higher than after noncardiac surgeries [49]. Additional prevention strategies have been considered (Table 8.10 [50]).

Table 8.10. Neuroprotective strategies in coronary artery bypass graft [50]

Timing	Issue	Intervention
Preoperative	Recognize risk factors	Neuropsychological testing
		Carotid ultrasonography
		MRI and MRA testing
	Atrial fibrillation	Pretreatment
Intraoperative	Aortic atheroma	Epiaortic ultrasound and TEE
		Avoid aortic clamping; minimize aortic manipulation and alteration of cannula placement
	Microemboli	Minimize cardiotomy suction and dissection of mediastinal fat
	Hypoperfusion	Maintain blood pressure during cardiopulmonary bypass
		Management with α-stat
	Brain hyperthermia	Avoid rapid and excessive rewarming
	Hyperglycemia	Avoid and treat hyperglycemia

MRI magnetic resonance imaging, *MRA* magnetic resonance angiography, *TEE* transthoracic echocardiography

References

1. Dyer CB, Ashton CM, Teasdale TA (1995) Postoperative delirium. A review of 80 primary data-collection studies. Arch Intern Med 155:461–465
2. Dasgupta M, Dumbrell AC (2006) Preoperative risk assessment for delirium after noncardiac surgery: a systematic review. J Am Geriatr Soc 54:1578–1589
3. Vochteloo AJ, Moerman S, van der Burg BL et al (2011) Delirium risk screening and haloperidol prophylaxis program in hip fracture patients is a helpful tool in identifying high-risk patients, but does not reduce the incidence of delirium. BMC Geriatr 11:39. doi:10.1186/1471-2318-11-39
4. Kalisvaart KJ, Vreeswijk R, de Jonghe JF et al (2006) Risk factors and prediction of postoperative delirium in elderly hip-surgery patients: implementation and validation of a medical risk factor model. J Am Geriatr Soc 54:817–822
5. Marcantonio ER, Goldman L, Mangione CM (1994) A clinical prediction rule for delirium after elective noncardiac surgery. JAMA 271:134–139
6. Ouimet S, Kavanagh BP, Gottfried SB et al (2007) Incidence, risk factors and consequences of ICU delirium. Intensive Care Med 33:66–73
7. Chaput AJ, Bryson GL (2012) Postoperative delirium: risk factors and management: continuing professional development. Can J Anaesth 59:304–320
8. Mason SE, Noel-Storr A, Ritchie CW (2010) The impact of general and regional anesthesia on the incidence of post-operative cognitive dysfunction and post-operative delirium: a systematic review with meta-analysis. J Alzheimers Dis 22:67–79
9. Nishikawa K, Nakayama M, Omote K et al (2004) Recovery characteristics and post-operative delirium after long-duration laparoscope-assisted surgery in elderly patients: propofol-based vs. sevoflurane-based anesthesia. Acta Anaesthesiol Scand 48:162–168
10. Sieber FE, Zakriya KJ, Gottschalk A et al (2010) Sedation depth during spinal anesthesia and the development of postoperative delirium in elderly patients undergoing hip fracture repair. Mayo Clin Proc 85:18–26
11. Radtke FM, Franck M, Lendner J et al (2013) Monitoring depth of anaesthesia in a randomized trial decreases the rate of postoperative delirium but not postoperative cognitive dysfunction. Br J Anaesth 110:i98–105

12. Mashour GA, Woodrum DT, Avidan MS (2015) Neurological complications of surgery and anaesthesia. Br J Anaesth 114:194–203
13. Nunomiya S (2012) Delirium. ICU & CCU 36:507–513
14. Marcantonio ER, Flacker JM, Wright RJ et al (2001) Reducing delirium after hip fracture: a randomized trial. J Am Geriatr Soc 49:516–522
15. Lundström M, Olofsson B, Stenvall M et al (2007) Postoperative delirium in old patients with femoral neck fracture: a randomized intervention study. Aging Clin Exp Res 19:178–186
16. Gosch M, Nicholas JA (2014) Pharmacologic prevention of postoperative delirium. Z Gerontol Geriatr 47:105–109
17. Wang W, Li HL, Wang DX et al (2012) Haloperidol prophylaxis decreases delirium incidence in elderly patients after noncardiac surgery: a randomized controlled trial. Crit Care Med 40:731–739
18. Prakanrattana U, Prapaitrakool S (2007) Efficacy of risperidone for prevention of postoperative delirium in cardiac surgery. Anaesth Intensive Care 35:714–719
19. Larsen KA, Kelly SE, Stern TA et al (2010) Administration of olanzapine to prevent postoperative delirium in elderly joint-replacement patients: a randomized, controlled trial. Psychosomatics 51:409–418
20. Aizawa K, Kanai T, Saikawa Y et al (2002) A novel approach to the prevention of postoperative delirium in the elderly after gastrointestinal surgery. Surg Today 32:310–314
21. Sultan SS (2010) Assessment of role of perioperative melatonin in prevention and treatment of postoperative delirium after hip arthroplasty under spinal anesthesia in the elderly. Saudi J Anaesth 4:169–173
22. Liptzin B, Laki A, Garb JL et al (2005) Donepezil in the prevention and treatment of post-surgical delirium. Am J Geriatr Psychiatry 13:1100–1106
23. Gamberini M, Bolliger D, Lurati Buse GA et al (2009) Rivastigmine for the prevention of postoperative delirium in elderly patients undergoing elective cardiac surgery—a randomized controlled trial. Crit Care Med 37:1762–1768
24. Leung JM, Sands LP, Rico M et al (2006) Pilot clinical trial of gabapentin to decrease postoperative delirium in older patients. Neurology 67:1251–1253
25. Radtke FM, Franck M, Lorenz M et al (2010) Remifentanil reduces the incidence of post-operative delirium. J Int Med Res 38:1225–1232
26. Pasin L, Landoni G, Nardelli P et al (2014) Dexmedetomidine reduces the risk of delirium, agitation and confusion in critically ill patients: a meta-analysis of randomized controlled trials. J Cardiothorac Vasc Anesth 28:1459–1466
27. Fok MC, Sepehry AA, Frisch L et al (2015) Do antipsychotics prevent postoperative delirium? A systematic review and meta-analysis. Int J Geriatr Psychiatry 30:333–344
28. Devlin JW, Roberts RJ, Fong JJ et al (2010) Efficacy and safety of quetiapine in critically ill patients with delirium: a prospective, multicenter, randomized, double-blind, placebo-controlled pilot study. Crit Care Med 38:419–427
29. van Eijk MM, Roes KC, Honing ML et al (2010) Effect of rivastigmine as an adjunct to usual care with haloperidol on duration of delirium and mortality in critically ill patients: a multicentre, double-blind, placebo-controlled randomised trial. Lancet 376:1829–1837
30. Moller JT, Cluitmans P, Rasmussen LS et al (1998) Long-term postoperative cognitive dysfunction in the elderly ISPOCD1 study. ISPOCD investigators. International study of post-operative cognitive dysfunction. Lancet 351:857–861
31. Abildstrom H, Rasmussen LS, Rentowl P et al (2000) Cognitive dysfunction 1-2 years after non-cardiac surgery in the elderly. ISPOCD group. International study of post-operative cognitive dysfunction. Acta Anaesthesiol Scand 44:1246–1251
32. Monk TG, Weldon BC, Garvan CW et al (2008) Predictors of cognitive dysfunction after major noncardiac surgery. Anesthesiology 108:18–30
33. Hudetz JA, Iqbal Z, Gandhi SD et al (2007) Postoperative cognitive dysfunction in older patients with a history of alcohol abuse. Anesthesiology 106:423–430
34. Hudetz JA, Patterson KM, Amole O et al (2011) Postoperative cognitive dysfunction after noncardiac surgery: effects of metabolic syndrome. J Anesth 25:337–344

35. Krenk L, Rasmussen LS, Kehlet H (2010) New insights into the pathophysiology of postoperative cognitive dysfunction. Acta Anaesthesiol Scand 54:951–956
36. Cibelli M, Fidalgo AR, Terrando N et al (2010) Role of interleukin-1beta in postoperative cognitive dysfunction. Ann Neurol 68:360–368
37. Hole A, Terjesen T, Breivik H (1980) Epidural versus general anaesthesia for total hip arthroplasty in elderly patients. Acta Anaesthesiol Scand 24:279–287
38. Evered L, Scott DA, Silbert B et al (2011) Postoperative cognitive dysfunction is independent of type of surgery and anesthetic. Anesth Analg 112:1179–1185
39. Hartholt KA, van der Cammen TJ, Klimek M (2012) Postoperative cognitive dysfunction in geriatric patients. Z Gerontol Geriatr 45:411–416
40. Tian A, Ma H, Cao X et al (2015) Vitamin D improves cognitive function and modulates Th17/T reg cell balance after hepatectomy in mice. Inflammation 38:500–509
41. Jin WJ, Feng SW, Feng Z et al (2014) Minocycline improves postoperative cognitive impairment in aged mice by inhibiting astrocytic activation. Neuroreport 25:1–6
42. Zhang J, Tan H, Jiang W et al (2014) Amantadine alleviates postoperative cognitive dysfunction possibly by increasing glial cell line-derived neurotrophic factor in rats. Anesthesiology 121:773–785
43. Kawano T, Takahashi T, Iwata H et al (2014) Effects of ketoprofen for prevention of postoperative cognitive dysfunction in aged rats. J Anesth 28:932–936
44. Sun D, Yang L, Wu Y et al (2014) Effect of intravenous infusion of dobutamine hydrochloride on the development of early postoperative cognitive dysfunction in elderly patients via inhibiting the release of tumor necrosis factor-α. Eur J Pharmacol 741:150–155
45. Tian Y, Zhao P, Li L et al (2014) Pre-emptive parecoxib and post-operative cognitive function in elderly patients. Int Psychogeriatr 15:1–8
46. Fang Q, Qian X, An J et al (2014) Higher dose dexamethasone increases early postoperative cognitive dysfunction. J Neurosurg Anesthesiol 26:220–225
47. Ottens TH, Dieleman JM, Sauër AM et al (2015) Effects of dexamethasone on cognitive decline after cardiac surgery: a randomized clinical trial. Anesthesiology 121:492–500
48. Sun JH, Wu XY, Wang WJ et al (2012) Cognitive dysfunction after off-pump versus on-pump coronary artery bypass surgery: a meta-analysis. J Int Med Res 40:852–858
49. van Harten AE, Scheeren TW, Absalom AR (2012) A review of postoperative cognitive dysfunction and neuroinflammation associated with cardiac surgery and anaesthesia. Anaesthesia 67:280–293
50. Goto T, Maekawa K (2014) Cerebral dysfunction after coronary artery bypass surgery. J Anesth 28:242–248

Chapter 9
Mechanisms of POD and POCD: Effects of Anesthetics

Tomoyuki Miyazaki, Yoshikazu Yamaguchi, and Takahisa Goto

Abstract Postoperative delirium (POD) and postoperative cognitive dysfunction (POCD) worsen quality of life in postoperative patients and, moreover, impose huge cost on hospitals. Previous clinical reports revealed that POD appears to be a risk for high mortality in the elderly and POCD appears to have long-lasting adverse effect on learning performance in children. Nevertheless nobody has proposed the effective way to cure them. We are still struggling in exploring mechanisms underlying POD and POCD because of the following reasons: (1) clinical definitions may be obscure, (2) underlying mechanisms are multifactorial, (3) less animal models comparable with patients are available. Under these difficulties, a considerable number of studies have contributed to identify key molecules and neural circuits essential for the establishment of these diseases and fortunately some of them appear to postulate reliable mechanisms. Integrating latest findings, here we discuss about these mechanisms underlying POD and POCD.

Keywords POD • POCD • Acetylcholin • Monoamine • Orexin • Adenosine Melatonin • Amyloid beta • Caspase • Chloride transporter • AMPA receptor GABA receptor

9.1 The Pathogenesis Underlying Delirium

The etiology and pathogenesis of delirium are very complex and not entirely understood. The mechanism of general anesthetics is also in the middle of the process of elucidation. Currently, delirium is known to be a multifactorial disorder [1], and the

T. Miyazaki, M.D., Ph.D.
Department of Physiology/Anesthesiology, Graduate School of Medicine, Yokohama City University, 3-9 Fukuura, Kanazawa-ku, Yokohama, Kanagawa 236-0004, Japan
e-mail: johney4@hotmail.com

Y. Yamaguchi, M.D. • T. Goto, M.D., Ph.D.
Department of Anesthesiology, Graduate School of Medicine, Yokohama City University, 3-9 Fukuura, Kanazawa-ku, Yokohama, Kanagawa 236-0004, Japan

Y. Morimoto (ed.), *Anesthesia and Neurotoxicity*,
DOI 10.1007/978-4-431-55624-4_9

physiology of consciousness and wakefulness represents the results of a complex neural network and neurotransmitters.

The development of delirium in patients is the result of inter-relationships between predisposing factors and precipitating factors. Many mechanisms of delirium have been proposed and include neurotransmitter-, inflammation-, physiological stressor-, metabolic disorder-, and genetic factor-based mechanisms (Table 9.1) [2, 3].

Table 9.1 Potential pathophysiological contributors to delirium [2]

		Surgery		Intensive
	General medicine	Noncardiac	Cardiac	care unit
(a)				
Predisposing factors				
Dementia	2.3–4.7	2.8	–	–
Cognitive impairment	2.1–2.8	3.5–4.2	1.3	–
History of delirium	–	3.0	–	–
Functional impairment	4.0	2.5–3.5	–	–
Visual impairment	2.1–3.5	1.1–3.0	–	–
Hearing impairment	–	1.3	–	–
Comorbidity or severity of illness	1.3–5.6	4.3	–	1.1
Depression	3.2	–	1.2	–
History of transient ischemia or stroke	–	–	1.6	–
Alcohol misuse	5.7	1.4–3.3	–	–
Older age (≥75 years)	4.0	3.3–6.6	–	1.1
Precipitating factors				
Drugs				
Several drugs used	2.9	–	–	–
Psychoactive drugs	4.5	–	–	–
Sedatives or hypnotics	–	–	–	4.5
Use of physical restraints	3.2–4.4	–	–	–
Use of bladder catheter	2.4	–	–	–
Physiological				
Increased serum urea	5.1	–	–	1.1
Increased BUN:creatinine ratio	2.0	2.9	–	–
Abnormal serum albumin	–	–	1.4	–
Abnormal sodium, glucose, or potassium	–	3.4	–	–
Metabolic acidosis	–	–	–	1.4
Infection	–	–	–	3.1
Any iatrogenic event	1.9	–	–	–
Surgery				
Aortic aneurysm	–	8.3	–	–
Noncardiac thoracic	–	3.5	–	–
Neurosurgery	–	–	–	4.5
Trauma admission	–	–	–	3.4

Table 9.1 (continued)

	General medicine	Surgery		Intensive care unit
		Noncardiac	Cardiac	
Urgent admission	–	–	–	1.5
Coma	–	–	–	1.8–21.3
Data are relative risks. Some data are reported as ranges. The appendix contains a complete list of references				
BUN = blood urea nitrogen				
Risk factors for delirium from validated predictive models				

(b)

	Type of data available	*Review published*
Neurotransmitters		
Acetylcholine	Experimental and observational	Yes
Dopamine	Experimental and observational	Yes
γ-aminobutyric acid	Experimental and observational	No
Melatonin	Experimental and observational	Yes
Tryptophan or serotonin	Observational	Yes
Glutamate	Observational	No
Epinephrine or norepinephrine	Hypothetical	No
Proinflammatory markers		No
Interferon α or β	Experimental	Yes
Interleukin6	Observational	Yes
Interleukin8	Observational	Yes
Interleukin10	Observational	No
Tumor necrosis factor α	Hypothetical	Yes
Interleukin 1β	Hypothetical	Yes
Prostaglandin E	Hypothetical	Yes
Physiological stressors		No
Cortisol	Observational	No
S100β	Observational	No
Neopterin	Observational	No
Hypoxia	Observational	No
Metabolic disorders		No
Lactic acidosis	Experimental and observational	No
Hypoglycemia or hyperglycemia	Observational	No
IGF1	Observational	Yes
Hypercapnia	Hypothetical	Yes

(continued)

Table 9.1 (continued)

	General medicine	Surgery Noncardiac	Cardiac	Intensive care unit
Electrolyte disorders		No		
Sodium, calcium, magnesium	Experimental and observational	No		
Genetic factors				
Apolipoprotein E	Observational	Yes		
Glucocorticoid receptor	Observational	No		
Dopamine transporter or receptor	Observational	Yes		
Toll-like receptor 4	Hypothetical	No		

Experimental means that controlled data—e.g., from clinical trials or inference from unintended side effects in human beings, or both—are available
Observational means that only observational data are available in human beings
Hypothetical means that studies in human beings are not yet available to support the mechanism. The appendix contains a complete list of references
Potential pathophysiological contributors to delirium

Experimental indicates that controlled data, e.g., data from clinical trials, inferences from unintended side effects in human beings, or both, are available. Observational indicates that only observational human data are available. Hypothetical indicates that studies in human beings are not yet available to support the mechanism. The appendix contains a complete list of references.

Cholinergic deficiency and dopamine excess are thought to be linked to delirium [4] because anticholinergic medications and drugs used to treat Parkinson's disease are associated with delirium [5, 6]. However, the cholinesterase inhibitor rivastigmine does not decrease the duration of delirium and might increase mortality [7]. Hence, it is difficult to resolve delirium with any treatment based on a single neurotransmitter. Moreover, neurotransmitters have mutual influences on one another. Hatta et al. reported that ramelteon, a melatonin receptor agonist, exhibits a preventive effect on delirium [8].

It is also important to understand the basic neurophysiology of awake-sleep switching and circadian rhythms. First, we review the architecture and neurophysiology that are essential for understanding the pathophysiology underlying delirium. The effect of the cholinergic pathway on delirium has been found to be arrestive, which we more intensively discuss here. Second, we review the substances that are related to circadian rhythms because the disruption of circadian rhythms is thought to increase the incidence of delirium.

9.1.1 Neurophysiology

9.1.1.1 Ascending Arousal System

In 1949, Moruzzi and Magoun reported that the basic mechanism of wakefulness lies in the reticular activating system. Subsequent studies revealed that the key components of wakefulness are not in the reticular formation but in cell groups in the mesopontine junction. Currently, these pathways are recognized together as the ascending arousal system.

9.1.1.2 Ascending Arousal System Including Cholinergic Pathways

The ascending arousal system contains two major branches, i.e., the cholinergic pathway and other monoaminergic pathways. Acetylcholine-producing cell groups in the pedunculopontine tegmentum and laterodorsal tegmentum (PPT/LDT) project to a relay and the reticular nuclei of the thalamus [9]. These inputs facilitate neural input from the thalamus to the cerebral cortex (thalamocortical transmission, Fig. 9.1).

Acetylcholine plays crucial roles in the rapid eye movement (REM) sleep state in which cortical neurons begin to fire in patterns similar to those of the awake state, and the sleep state precedes the onset of wakefulness. Cholinergic neurons located in the nucleus basalis of Meynert and the midbrain extend their axons all over the cerebral cortex and release acetylcholine locally from their presynaptic terminals immediately prior to the initiation of the REM sleep state. Locally released acetylcholine can desynchronize the firing patterns of cortical neurons, and the EEGs (electroencephalograms) generated by these neurons then increase in frequency and decrease in amplitude. These changes ready the cortical neurons for stimuli coming from other brain regions and ultimately led to consciousness. Cholinergic activity also correlates with cognitive function in laboratory animals [11, 12]. The administration of high-dose atropine to animals increases the total serum anticholinergic activity in a dose-dependent manner [13]. Biperiden, which is another type of

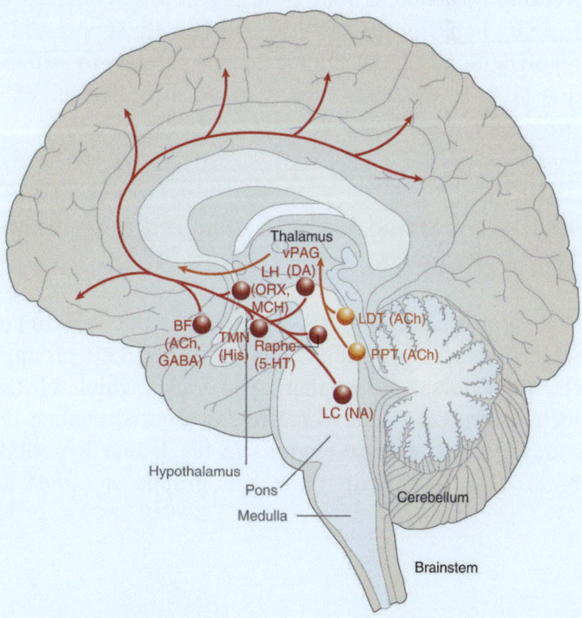

Fig. 9.1 Schematic drawing of the ascending arousal system [10]

anticholinergic drug, induces behavioral and polygraphic changes similar to those of delirious patients who can be observed on electroencephalography, electrooculography, and electromyography [14]. These findings are also true in delirious patients whose serum anticholinergic activities are significantly greater than those of nondelirious patients [15]. Moreover, drug-induced dysfunction of the cholinergic pathway produces delirium and disorientation [16]. Based on accumulating evidence suggesting the positive effect of acetylcholine on cognitive function, the pharmacological regulation of the cholinergic pathway had been intensively studied as a therapeutic target in dementia patients. Actually, drugs that increase the acetylcholine concentration by inhibiting acetylcholine esterase have been used in clinical settings.

In addition to the enhancing effect of acetylcholine on cognition, an inhibitory effect of acetylcholine on attention has recently been identified [17]. As mentioned above, acetylcholine works as a neurotransmitter and binds to two types of receptor, i.e., muscarinic and nicotinic. While antagonism of the muscarinic receptors reduces attention, antagonism of the nicotinic receptors has no effect [18]. By definition, delirium includes reduced awareness. Therefore, delirious states result can be understood to result from a lack of attention rather than a lack of cognition. In laboratory animals, several behavioral tests are available to elucidate the effects of anesthetic agents on attention. The latent inhibition test is a major test of attentional ability. In this test, mice are divided into two groups, e.g., a pre-exposed group (the mice are exposed to 40 white noise tones of 5 s in duration with an inter-noise interval of 25 s) and a non-pre-exposed group. On the first day, immediately after pre-exposure to the tone, the mice experience tone–shock pairing. On the day 3, the mice are moved to a new space and allowed to explore for 180 sec, followed by exposure to the tone for 180 s, and the experimenters then measure the durations of freezing behavior in both groups. If a mouse attends to the tone on the first day, freezing behavior on day 3 is significantly suppressed and vice versa. A previous report demonstrated that mice that are exposed to isoflurane exhibit decreased attention [19]. In contrast, mice exposed to desflurane exhibit no effect on attention (Miyazaki, submitted).

9.1.1.3 Ascending Arousal System Including the Monoaminergic Pathways

The monoaminergic pathways include the tuberomammillary nucleus (TMN), which releases histamine (His), the A10 cell group, which releases dopamine (DA), the dorsal and median raphe nuclei, which release serotonin (5-HT), and the locus coeruleus (LC), which releases noradrenaline (NA) (Fig. 9.1). These neurotransmitters activate neurons in the lateral hypothalamic area and basal forebrain. The neurons in these cell groups are most active during wakefulness, exhibited decreased activity during non-REM sleep, and are silent during REM sleep [20, 21].

9.1.1.4 Sleep-Promoting System

Whereas the ascending arousal system is the key region for the maintenance of wakeful states, the neurons located in the ventrolateral preoptic nuclei (VLPO) and median preoptic nuclei (MnPO) are key to the promotion of sleep states. The VLPO provides inhibitory GABAergic and galaninergic outputs to the TMN and other regions of the ascending arousal system [22]. γ-aminobutyric acid (GABA) is the major inhibitory neurotransmitter. Cell-specific lesions of the VLPO in animals reduce NREM and REM sleep by more than 50% [23, 24]. Lesions of the VLPO cluster reduce NREM sleep, although lesions of the extended VLPO disrupt REM sleep. These findings indicate that GABA release from the VLPO is crucial to driving sleep states (Fig. 9.2).

Recent studies have revealed that dexmedetomidine reduces the duration of postoperative delirium compared with propofol [25]. The guidelines suggest that dexmedetomidine infusions that are administered for sedation may be associated with a lower prevalence of delirium compared with benzodiazepine infusions [26]. The

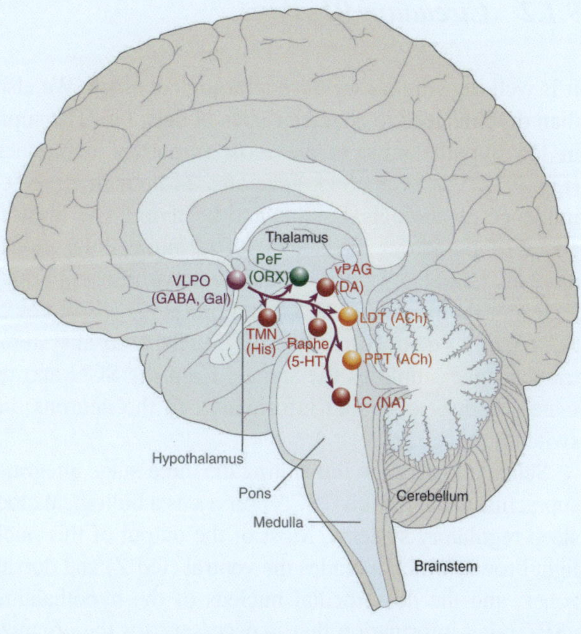

Fig. 9.2 Schematic drawing of the relationship between the VLPO and the ascending arousal system [10]

postoperative plasma GABA concentration is associated with postoperative delirium in critically ill patients [27].

9.1.1.5 The Flip-Flop System and Orexin Neurons

Although we spend one-third of our lives asleep, the sleep-wake switching mechanism requires only a few seconds to a minute. Sleep-wake switching is the result of a reciprocal relationship between the VLPO and the ascending arousal system. Saper et al. suggested that this relationship is like a "flip-flop." The two halves of the flip-flop circuit create a feedback loop that is bistable via mutual inhibition; i.e., there are two possible stable firing patterns, and intermediate states tend to be avoided [28]. Orexin neurons play an important role in stabilizing this system. A single study reported the relationship between general anesthesia and orexin. The plasma orexin A level is increased 5 min after extubation compared with the level following anesthetic induction [29]. It is unclear how orexin affects postoperative delirium and postoperative cognitive dysfunction. Suvorexant, which is a novel dual antagonist of the OX1R and OX2R orexin receptors, is receiving attention as the novel therapy for insomnia. However, its use should be closely monitored in patients who are at risk for delirium [30].

9.1.2 Circadian Rhythms

It is well known that we have a biological clock. We also know that impaired circadian rhythms lead to characteristics of delirium. The suprachiasmatic nucleus (SCN) in the hypothalamus is the most important component of the biological clock (Fig. 9.3). The SCN clock generates 24-hour rhythms (e.g., circadian rhythms) that influence physiological status and behavior. The master clock in the SCN is composed of numerous clock cells. The intracellular clock mechanism in the mouse involves interacting positive and negative transcriptional feedback loops that drive recurrent rhythms in the RNA and protein levels of key clock components [31]. The SCN neurons do not directly project to the arousal system or VLPO. The subparaventricular zone amplifies the signals from the SCN and dorsomedial nucleus to ultimately convey circadian information to the neurons that control wake-sleep state switching [10, 32].

Schematic diagram illustrating the three-stage integrator of circadian rhythms. The suprachiasmatic nucleus (SCN) serves as a biological clock but has few outputs to the sleep-regulatory systems. Most of the output of this nucleus goes into the region in light brown, which includes the ventral (vSPZ) and dorsal (dSPZ) subparaventricular zones, and the dorsomedial nucleus of the hypothalamus (DMH). Neurons in the vSPZ relay information that is necessary for the organization of the daily cycles of wake–sleep, whereas the dSPZ neurons are crucial for rhythms in body temperature.

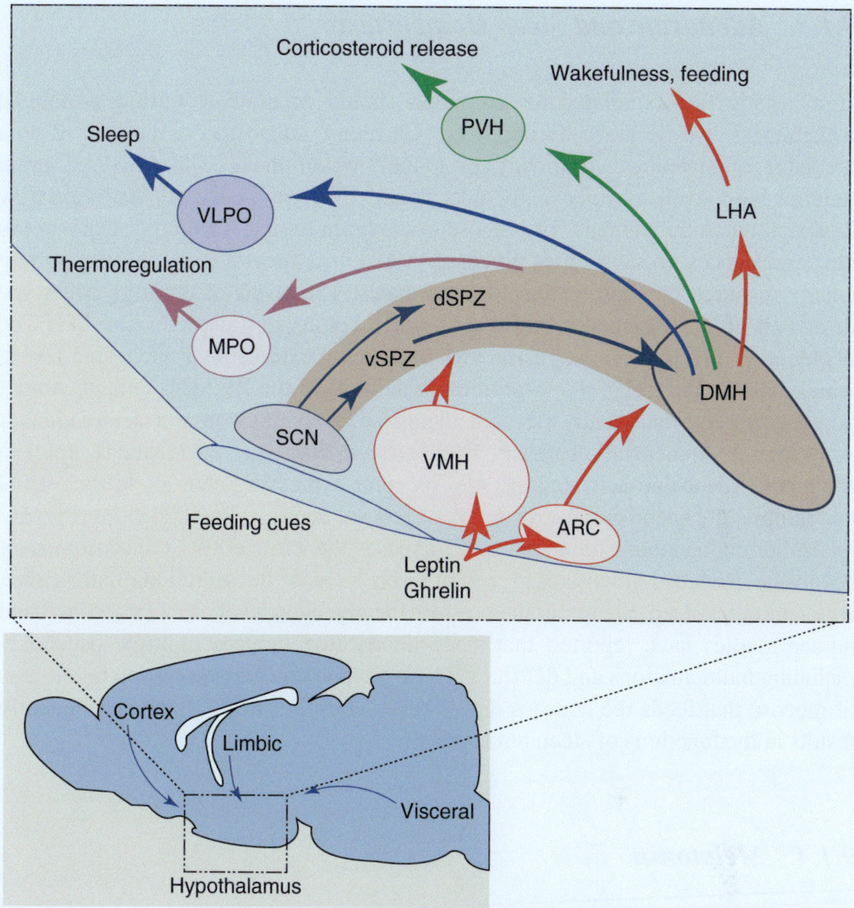

Fig. 9.3 Neural circuit that promotes circadian rhythms [10]

In the DMH, the outputs from the SPZ are integrated with other inputs, and DMH neurons drive the circadian cycles of sleep, activity, feeding, and corticosteroid secretion. Cycles in body temperature are maintained by the dSPZ projections back to the medial preoptic area (MPO), whereas the DMN is the origin of projections to the VLPO that regulate sleep cycles, projections to the corticotropin-releasing hormone (CRH) neurons of the paraventricular nucleus (PVH) that regulate corticosteroid cycles, and projections to the lateral hypothalamic (LHA) orexin and melanin-concentrating hormone neurons that regulate wakefulness and feeding cycles. The integrative steps in the SPZ and DMH allow circadian rhythms to adapt to environmental stimuli, such as food availability (e.g., the action of leptin and ghrelin via the ventromedial (VMH) and arcuate (ARC) nuclei), as well as visceral sensory inputs, cognitive influences from the prefrontal cortex, and emotional inputs from the limbic system (inset).

9.1.3 Adenosine and Sleep Homeostasis

Homeostatic factors related to sleepiness should accumulate during prolonged wakefulness and decrease during sleep. Currently, adenosine is recognized as a mediator of sleepiness following prolonged wakefulness. The activated brain requires high levels of glucose, but occasionally the glucose supply via blood flow does not match the demand for glucose in the brain during learning or exposure to new experiences. In such cases, glycogen stored in astrocytes is the most important energy resource for these activated brain states. The levels of brain glycogen are decreased after prolonged wakefulness, which results in a depletion of ATP. The depletion of glycogen causes astrocytes to increase extracellular adenosine levels, which inhibits the wakefulness-promoting neurons in the BF [33]. This phenomenon may suggest that locally elevated adenosine levels function as a sleep indicator that monitors homeostatic balance. There are two classes of adenosine receptor in the brain. Adenosine activates the A2a receptor-expressing neurons in the VLPO and inhibits the adenosine A1 receptors of arousal neurons. Prostaglandin (PG) D2 is also an endogenous somnogen that increases the extracellular concentration of adenosine. Reduced glucose or glycogen levels increase the secretion of adenosine, which initiates sleep. Sleep can then restore the glycogen level. Previous animal and human studies have reported that sleep deprivation induces multiple psychoses including hallucinations and delirium. These phenomena may be caused by the loss of glucose that feeds the neurons that regulate consciousness, which subsequently results in dysfunctions of sleep homeostasis.

9.1.4 Melatonin

Melatonin is secreted from the pineal gland at night and is an important hormone for the maintenance of circadian rhythm and affects many organs. The secretion of melatonin is subject to the control of the SCN [34] and is affected by sunlight. Melatonin is also commercially available as a drug that improves insomnia. This fact supports the notion that melatonin is a key player in the control of circadian rhythms. Interestingly ketamine and pentobarbital affect circadian rhythms in a different manner via the production of phase delays or advances in pineal melatonin secretion, and these changes cause abnormal locomotor activity [35].

9.2 The Pathogenesis Underlying POCD

In contrast to postoperative delirium, the definition of postoperative cognitive dysfunction (POCD) is unclear. Thus, the prevalence of POCD is also currently unclear, which prevents us from exploring the mechanism underlying POCD. Therefore, it is difficult to elucidate the direct relationships between exposure to anesthetic agents and cognitive dysfunction in clinical settings because a patient is subjected to both anesthesia and surgical invasion during an operation. A previous animal study demonstrated that surgery with local anesthesia (without general anesthesia) induces POCD in elderly but not adult mice via the accumulation of amyloid beta [36], which indicates that a surgical insult is sufficient to cause cognitive dysfunction. However, accumulating evidence indicates that exposure to anesthetic agents alone induces cognitive dysfunction, at least in laboratory animals including mice, rats, and monkeys [37, 38]. A considerable number of studies have demonstrated that the effects of anesthesia on POCD vary depending on the following factors: (1) the type of anesthetic agent, (2) the exposure concentration, (3) the duration of exposure, and (4) the number of days between the exposure to anesthesia and cognitive testing. We usually perform multiple tests to comprehensively study cognitive functions in rodents. For example, place memory is coded in the hippocampus [39], and emotional memory is partially coded in the amygdala [40]. Our original animal data suggest that isoflurane decreases attention [19], whereas sevoflurane exerts an antidepressive effect (preliminary data). These effects have also been confirmed at anesthetic concentrations above 1 MAC, which indicates dose-dependent effects. However, why the effects of different anesthetic agents on behavioral phenotype vary widely remains unclear. To some extent, these differences can be accounted for by the expression patterns of the target receptors to which the anesthetic agents bind (Fig. 9.4) [41]. Regarding the duration of anesthetic exposure, longer exposures can elicit worse effects on learning performance. Regarding the duration of these effects, the age at which the animals are exposed to the anesthetic agents is crucial; the

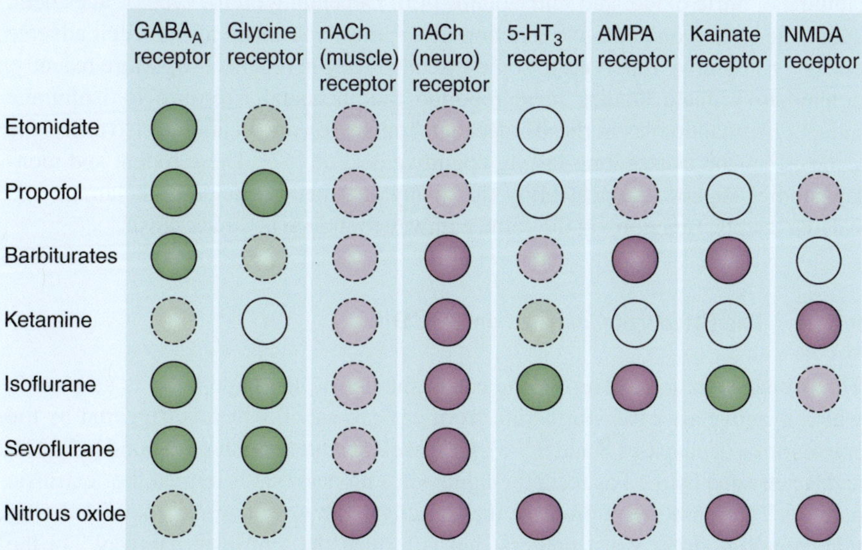

Fig. 9.4 Effects of general anesthetics on ligand-gated ion channels

effects of anesthesia on cognitive function vary widely between neonate, adult, and elderly animals. In juveniles and adults, these adverse effects of anesthetic agents never seem to last more than a month [42]. Although these adverse effects may occasionally be neglected in juveniles and adults, the effects of anesthetic exposure on neonates are gradually exacerbated. Among the four above-mentioned factors, the effects of age at the time of exposure to anesthetic agents are the worthiest of focus. Here, we summarize the effects of anesthesia on POCD in terms of age and clarify the factors that cause POCD in each age group.

9.2.1 Effects in Neonates

The effects of anesthesia on cognitive function in neonates have been the most extensively studied thus far. Neonatal animals are susceptible to external factors because neural circuits exhibit rapid development during the neonatal period. Neonatal neurons are so plastic that exposure to drugs, stress, and other manipulations can easily modify the expressions or functions of key molecules that regulate cognition and emotion, and these modifications are long lasting and occasionally irreversible [43]. Ikonomidou published the first report to examining the relationship between anesthetic agents and cognitive function. This paper revealed that NMDA receptor antagonists function in a manner similar to ketamine to cause widespread apoptotic neurodegeneration in neonatal rat brains that is followed by learning impairments in the adults [44]. Todorovic et al. also reported that the same phenomenon can be induced by volatile anesthetics (i.e., mixed agents including isoflurane, nitric oxide, and midazolam) [45]. Depending on the type of anesthetic agent, the effects on cognitive function differ; most anesthetic agents elicit adverse effects on cognitive functions to some extent, at least in rodents [46]. More recently, nonhuman primate studies have reported that neonatal exposure to isoflurane induces neuroapoptosis in rhesus macaque brains [38], and ketamine also exerts the same effect and causes long-lasting cognitive decline [47]. These rodent and monkey studies suggest the possibility that many anesthetics, including ketamine and volatile agents, function via the same pathway to induce neuroapoptosis.

9.2.1.1 The Effects of Caspases on POCD

The primary factor involved in the establishment of neuroapoptosis is caspase 3, which is active after transformation from pro-caspase 3, which is triggered by the active forms of caspases 8 and 9 [48]. Caspase 8 is a protease that is bound to FADD and is activated by the Fas receptor signal via a process that is termed the "extrinsic pathway." Caspase 9 is a protease that is activated by cytochrome c/apaf-1 during mitochondrial stress via a process that is termed the "intrinsic pathway." In the recent few years, the regulation of caspase activity has received attention as promising target for the treatment of POCD. The administrations of erythropoietin, estradiol, melatonin, and dexmedetomidine have been reported to improve anesthesia-induced neuroapoptosis [49–52] via the deactivation of caspase activity. Hydrogen gas has also been proven to reduce caspase 3 activity and neuroapoptosis and induce a subsequent attenuation of learning impairment in the adult [53]. Interestingly, the same group reported that the exposure of female pups to desflurane induces the maltreatment of pups after the exposed animals become mothers, and hydrogen gas also rescues this maternal care [54].

9.2.1.2 The Effect of NKCC1/KCC2 on POCD

The overexcitation of neurons also leads to neuronal death. Koyama and we have studied the effects of midazolam and propofol on the function of the chloride transporter in the neonate [55]. NKCC1 is the neonatal subunit of chloride ion transporter and is dominant over KCC2 in the neonate. NKCC1 maintains the intracellular chloride ion concentration at a level greater than the extracellular concentration. Under this condition, GABAA receptor activators, including midazolam and propofol, open chloride channels, which leads to chloride ion efflux and subsequent neuronal depolarization, which in turn leads to the overexcitation of neurons (Fig. 9.5). This process precedes neuroapoptosis, but the induction of neuroapoptosis can be rescued via the inactivation of NKCC1. We have also demonstrated that the NKCC1 blocker bumetanide attenuates anesthetic-induced neuronal hyperexcitability.

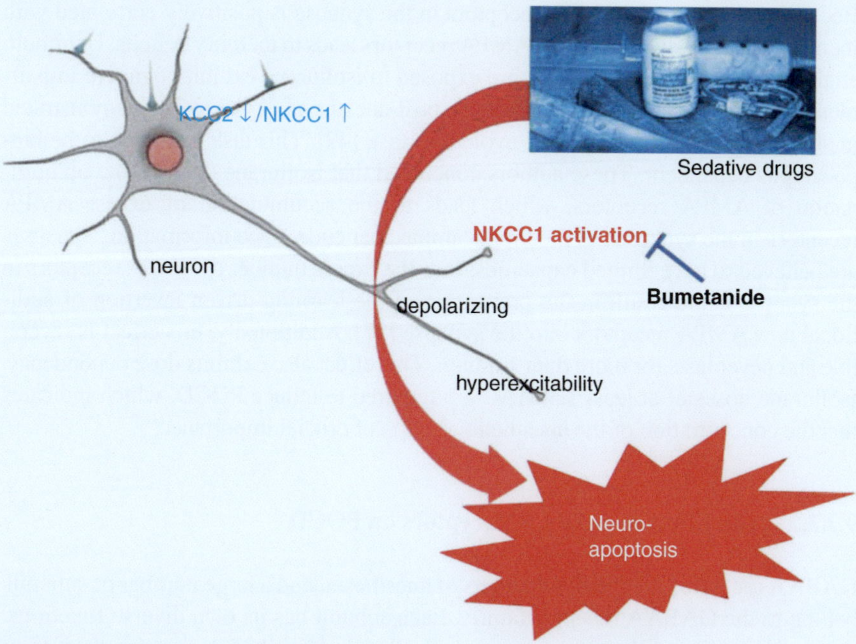

Fig. 9.5 The effect of chloride ion transporter on neuroapoptosis

However, bumetanide also functions as a diuretic and is not suitable for clinical use. Recently, Gagnon succeeded in producing a KCC2 activator [56] that is fascinating in terms of its ability to regulate neuronal excitability.

9.2.2 *Effects in Adults*

As described above, neonates are highly plastic and susceptible to external factors. Thus, the effects of anesthesia may last for extended periods. Although adult animals are believed to have previously established neural circuits that exhibit resistance to external factors, some studies have demonstrated anesthesia-induced cognitive dysfunction in adults. There are numerous key molecules that modify neuronal function, and most of these molecules ultimately affect excitatory or inhibitory receptors to maintain the balance between the excitation and inhibition of neurons. Excitation is primarily controlled by α-amino-3-hydroxy-5-methyl-4-isoxazolepropionic acid (AMPA) receptors, and inhibition is primarily controlled by GABAA receptors. The disruption of the inhibition-excitation balance weakens synaptic connectivity and neural circuits, and animals subsequently exhibit deficiencies in learning and memory.

9.2.2.1 The Effects of AMPA Receptors on POCD

Because the number of AMPA receptors in the synapse is positively correlated with memory strength, dysfunction of AMPA receptors leads to memory deficits. Uchimoto et al. reported that adult rats that are exposed to isoflurane exhibit cognitive impairments in terms of place information from post-anesthesia days 3 to 7 as demonstrated in studies utilizing the inhibitory avoidance task [42]. This task is known to be hippocampus dependent. These authors concluded that isoflurane disturbs the ubiquitination of AMPA receptors, which leads to the accumulation of excess AMPA receptors in the synapses of the hippocampus that code place information. Synapses are believed to have limited capacities; thus the excess number of AMPA receptors in the synapse could result in the prevention of the learning-driven insertion of additional new AMPA receptors into the synapse [57]. Additionally, this effect is reversible and never lasts for more than 1 month. This effect also exhibits dose dependency. Isoflurane doses of at least 1.3 MAC are required to induce POCD, which indicates that the concentration of the anesthetic agent is of crucial importance.

9.2.2.2 The Effect of GABAA Receptors on POCD

GABAA receptors are the main targets of anesthesia, and a large number of subunits belong to the GABAA receptor family. Each subunit has its own diverse functions. Saab et al. reported that an exposure to isoflurane of only 1 h impairs short-term memory. Interestingly, the administration of an alfa5 GABAA receptor inverse agonist rescues this effect [58]. The same effect is also exerted by etomidate via the targeting of the alfa5 GABAA receptor [59]. Although many studies have revealed adverse effects of anesthesia on cognitive function in adults, some have demonstrated the absence of this effect or even the opposite effect. Stratmann et al. reported that isoflurane does not affect long-term cognitive function. Additionally, Hauer et al. reported that propofol elicits a positive effect on cognitive function 2 days after its administration that is mediated by an enhancement of the endogenous cannabinoid system [60].

9.2.3 *Effects in the Elderly*

Particularly in the elderly, the maintenance of neuronal homeostasis can be difficult. To retain cell viability, the maintenance of a stable membrane potential is essential. Membrane proteins, including glycoproteins and ion channels, are frequently mobile on the surface of the plasma membrane in a manner that is ATP dependent, and these proteins play crucial roles in maintaining the membrane potential. Anesthetic agents prevent the mobility of these proteins and disturb the stability of the membrane potential. For example, an inappropriate membrane potential activates some types of calcium channels, which subsequently induces the initiation of calcium toxicity [61]. This sequence causes neuronal hyperexcitability and leads to the disruption of neuronal homeostasis and cell viability. Furthermore, excessive influx of calcium increases caspase activity, which leads to neuroapoptosis [62]. The functions of membrane proteins are directly and indirectly affected by anesthetic agents. The direct effect is mediated by the prevention of protein mobility due to the movement of the anesthetic compounds into plasma membrane, which increases the volume. The indirect effect is mediated by a reduction in blood flow followed by reductions in oxygen and glucose delivery that prevent ATP-dependent membrane protein mobility.

9.2.3.1 The Effect of Anesthetics on the Synthesis of Amyloid Beta

Amyloid beta has been intensively studied as a key factor in the establishment of Alzheimer's disease. Alzheimer's disease patients exhibit progressive cognitive dysfunction. One of the most evident mechanisms underlying Alzheimer disease is the accumulation of amyloid beta in neurons, which prevents new protein synthesis that is essential for cell viability. Xie et al. reported that exposure to isoflurane at 1.4% for 2 h promotes the accumulation of amyloid beta and increases caspasc 3 activity in micc [63]. Lu et al. also reported that exposure to sevoflurane at 3.0% for 6 h promotes the accumulation of amyloid beta, increases caspase 3 activity, and induces neuroapoptosis in neonatal mice [64]. This effect is not observed in mice that are exposed to 3% sevoflurane for 2 h, which suggests a time-dependent mechanism. Moreover, the exposure of model mice with amyloid beta to sevoflurane also enhances the accumulation of amyloid beta.

References

1. Inouye SK, Charpentier PA (1996) Precipitating factors for delirium in hospitalized elderly persons. Predictive model and interrelationship with baseline vulnerability. JAMA 275:852–857
2. Inouye SK, Westendorp RG, Saczynski JS (2014) Delirium in elderly people. Lancet 383:911–922
3. Inouye SK, Westendorp RG, Saczynski JS, Kimchi EY, Cleinman AA (2014) Delirium in elderly people—authors' reply. Lancet 383:2045
4. Hshieh TT, Fong TG, Marcantonio ER, Inouye SK (2008) Cholinergic deficiency hypothesis in delirium: a synthesis of current evidence. J Gerontol A Biol Sci Med Sci 63:764–772
5. Han L, McCusker J, Cole M, Abrahamowicz M, Primeau F, Elie M (2001) Use of medications with anticholinergic effect predicts clinical severity of delirium symptoms in older medical inpatients. Arch Intern Med 161:1099–1105
6. Young BK, Camicioli R, Ganzini L (1997) Neuropsychiatric adverse effects of antiparkinsonian drugs. Characteristics, evaluation and treatment. Drugs Aging 10:367–383
7. Gamberini M, Bolliger D, Lurati Buse GA et al (2009) Rivastigmine for the prevention of postoperative delirium in elderly patients undergoing elective cardiac surgery--a randomized controlled trial. Crit Care Med 37:1762–1768
8. Hatta K, Kishi Y, Wada K et al (2014) Preventive effects of ramelteon on delirium: a randomized placebo-controlled trial. JAMA Psychiat 71:397–403
9. Hallanger AE, Levey AI, Lee HJ, Rye DB, Wainer BH (1987) The origins of cholinergic and other subcortical afferents to the thalamus in the rat. J Comp Neurol 262:105–124
10. Saper CB, Scammell TE, Lu J (2005) Hypothalamic regulation of sleep and circadian rhythms. Nature 437:1257–1263
11. Leavitt ML, Trzepacz PT, Ciongoli K et al (1994) Rat model of delirium: atropine dose–response relationships. J Neuropsychiatry Clin Neurosci 6:279–284
12. Trzepacz PT, Leavitt M, Ciongoli K (1992) An animal model for delirium. Psychosomatics 33:404–415
13. O'hare E, Welcon DT, Bettin K et al (1997) Serum anticholinergic activity and behavior following atropine sulfate administration in the rat. Pharmacol Biochem Behav 56:151–154
14. Tamura Y, Chiba S, Takasaki H et al (2006) Biperiden-induced delirium model in rats: a behavioral and electroencephalographic study. Brain Res 1115:194–199
15. Mach JR, Dysken MW, Kuskowski M et al (1995) Serum anticholinergic activity in hospitalized older persons with delirium: a preliminary study. J Am Geriatr Soc 43:491–495
16. Brown JH (1990) Atropine, scopolamine, and other related antimuscarinic drugs. In: Gilman AG, Rall TW, Nies AS, Taylor P (eds) The pharmacological basis of therapeutics. Pergamon Press, New York, pp 150–165
17. Klinkenberg I, Sambeth A, Blokland A (2011) Acetylcholine and attention. Behav Brain Res 221:430–442
18. Herrero JL, Roberts MJ, Delicato LS et al (2008) Acetylcholine contributes through muscarinic receptors to attentional modulation in V1. Nature 454:1110–1114
19. Yonezaki K, Uchimoto K, Miyazaki T et al (2015) Postanesthetic effects of isoflurane on behavioral phenotypes of adult male C57BL/6J mice. PLoS One 10:e0122118
20. Aston-Jones G, Bloom FE (1981) Activity of norepinephrine-containing locus coeruleus neurons in behaving rats anticipates fluctuations in the sleep-waking cycle. J Neurosci 1:876–886
21. Takahashi K, Kayama Y, Lin JS, Sakai K (2010) Locus coeruleus neuronal activity during the sleep-waking cycle in mice. Neuroscience 169:1115–1126
22. Sherin JE, Elmquist JK, Torrealba F, Saper CB (1998) Innervation of histaminergic tuberomammillary neurons by GABAergic and galaninergic neurons in the ventrolateral preoptic nucleus of the rat. J Neurosci 18:4705–4721
23. Lu J, Bjorkum AA, Xu M, Gaus SE, Shiromani PJ, Saper CB (2002) Selective activation of the extended ventrolateral preoptic nucleus during rapid eye movement sleep. J Neurosci 22:4568–4576

24. Lu J, Greco MA, Shiromani P, Saper CB (2000) Effect of lesions of the ventrolateral preoptic nucleus on NREM and REM sleep. J Neurosci 20:3830–3842
25. Djaiani G, Silverton N, Fedorko L et al (2016) Dexmedetomidine versus propofol sedation reduces delirium after cardiac surgery: a randomized controlled trial. Anesthesiology 124(2): 362–368
26. Barr J, Fraser GL, Puntillo K et al (2013) Clinical practice guidelines for the management of pain, agitation, and delirium in adult patients in the intensive care unit. Crit Care Med 41:263–306
27. Yoshitaka S, Egi M, Kanazawa T, Toda Y, Morita K (2014) The association of plasma gamma-aminobutyric acid concentration with postoperative delirium in critically ill patients. Crit Care Resusc 16:269–273
28. Saper CB, Chou TC, Scammell TE (2001) The sleep switch: hypothalamic control of sleep and wakefulness. Trends Neurosci 24:726–731
29. Wang ZH, Ni XL, Li JN et al (2014) Changes in plasma orexin-a levels in sevoflurane-remifentanil anesthesia in young and elderly patients undergoing elective lumbar surgery. Anesth Analg 118:818–822
30. Howland RH (2014) Suvorexant: a novel therapy for the treatment of insomnia. J Psychosoc Nurs Ment Health Serv 52:23–26
31. Reppert SM, Weaver DR (2002) Coordination of circadian timing in mammals. Nature 418:935–941
32. Saper CB, Fuller PM, Pedersen NP, Lu J, Scammell TE (2010) Sleep state switching. Neuron 68:1023–1042
33. Strecker RE, Morairty S, Thakkar MM et al (2000) Adenosinergic modulation of basal forebrain and preoptic/anterior hypothalamic neuronal activity in the control of behavioral state. Behav Brain Res 115:183–204
34. Pevet P, Challet E (2011) Melatonin: both master clock output and internal time-giver in the circadian clocks network. J Physiol Paris 105:170–182
35. Mihara T, Kikuchi T, Kamiya Y et al (2012) Day or night administration of ketamine and pentobarbital differentially affect circadian rhythms of pineal melatonin secretion and locomotor activity in rats. Anesth Analg 115:805–813
36. Xu Z, Dong Y, Culley DJ, Marcantonio ER, Crosby G, Tanzi RE, Zhang Y, Xie Z (2014) Age-dependent postoperative cognitive impairment and Alzheimer-related neuropathology in mice. Sci Rep 4:3766
37. Culley DJ, Baxter MG, Yukhananov R, Crosby G (2004) Long-term impairment of acquisition of a spatial memory task following isoflurane-nitrous oxide anesthesia in rats. Anesthesiology 100:309–314
38. Brambrink AM, Evers AS, Avidan MS, Farber NB, Smith DJ, Zhang X, Dissen GA, Creeley CE, Olney JW (2010) Isoflurane-induced neuroapoptosis in the neonatal rhesus macaque brain. Anesthesiology 112:834–841
39. Eichenbaum H, Dudchenko P, Wood E et al (1999) The hippocampus, memory, and place cells. Neuron 23:209–226
40. Cahill L, Babinsky R, Markowitsch R et al (1995) The amygdala and emotional memory. Nature 377:295–296
41. Rudolph U, Antkowtak B (2004) Molecular and neuronal substrate for general anesthetics. Nat Rev Neurosci 5:709–720
42. Uchimoto K, Miyazaki T, Kamiya Y et al (2014) Isoflurane impairs learning and hippocampal long-term potentiation via the saturation of synaptic plasticity. Anesthesiology 121: 302–310
43. Miyazaki T, Takase K, Nakajima W et al (2012) Disrupted cortical function underlies behavior dysfunction due to social isolation. J Clin Invest 122:2690–2701
44. Ikonomidou C, Bosch F, Miksa M et al (1999) Blockade of NMDA receptors and apoptotic neurodegeneration in the developing brain. Science 283:70–74
45. Jevtovic-Todorovic V, Hartman RE, Izumi Y et al (2003) Early exposure to common anesthetic agents causes widespread neurodegeneration in the developing rat brain and persistent learning deficits. J Neurosci 23:876–882

46. Jevtovic-Todorovic V, Absalom AR, Blomgren K et al (2013) Anaesthetic neurotoxicity and neuroplasticity: an expert group report and statement based on the BJA Salzburg seminar. BJA 111:143–151
47. Paule MG, Li M, Allen RR et al (2011) Ketamine anesthesia during the first week of life can cause long-lasting cognitive deficits in rhesus monkeys. Neurotoxicol Teratol 33:220–230
48. Goyal L (2001) Cell death inhibition: keeping caspases in check. Cell 104:805–808
49. Pellegrini L, Bennis Y, Velly L et al (2014) Erythropoietin protects newborn rat against sevoflurane-induced neurotoxicity. Pediat Anesth 24:749–759
50. Lu LX, Yon JH, Carter LB et al (2006) General anesthesia activates BDNF-dependent neuroapoptosis in the developing rat brain. Apoptosis 11:1603–1615
51. Yon JH, Carter LB, Reiter RJ et al (2006) Melatonin reduces the severity of anesthesia-induced apoptotic neurodegeneration in the developing rat brain. Nuerobiol Dis 21:522–530
52. Li Y, Zheg M, Chen W et al (2014) Dexmedetomidine reduces isoflurane-induced neuroapoptosis partly by preserving PI3K/Akt pathway in the hippocampus of neonatal rats. PLoS One 9(4):e93639
53. Yonamine R, Satoh Y, Kodama M et al (2013) Coadministration of hydrogen gas as part of the carrier gas mixture suppresses neuronal apoptosis and subsequent behavioral deficits caused by neonatal exposure to sevoflurane in mice. Anesthesiology 118:105–113
54. Takaenoki Y, Satoh Y, Araki Y et al (2014) Neonatal exposure to sevoflurane in mice causes deficits in maternal behavior later in adulthood. Anesthesiology 120:403–415
55. Koyama Y, Andoh T, Kamiya Y et al (2013) Bumetanide, an inhibitor of cation-chloride cotransporter isoform 1, inhibits gamma-aminobutyric acidergic excitatory actions and enhances sedative actions of midazolam in neonatal rats. Anesthesiology 119:1096–1108
56. Gagnon M, Bergeron MJ, Lavertu G et al (2013) Chloride extrusion enhancers as novel therapeutics for neurological diseases. Nat Med 19:1524–1528
57. Moser EI, Krobert KA, Moser MB et al (1998) Impaired spatial learning after saturation of long-term potentiation. Science 281:2038–2042
58. Saab BJ, Maclean AJ, Kanisek M et al (2010) Short-term memory impairment after isoflurane in mice is prevented by the alfa5 gamma-aminobutyric acid type a receptor inverse agonist L-655,708. Anesthesiology 113:1061–1071
59. Martin LJ, Oh GH, Orser BA (2009) Etomidate targets alpha5 gamma-aminobutyric acid subtype a receptors to regulate synaptic plasticity and memory blockade. Anesthesiology 111: 1025–1035
60. Hauer D, Ratano P, Morena M et al (2011) Propofol enhances memory formation Vis an interaction with the endocannabinoid system. Anesthesiology 114:1380–1388
61. Gagnon M, Siesjo BK (1992) Pathophysiology and treatment of focal cerebral ischemia. J Neurosurg 77:169–184
62. Dirnagi U, Iadecola C, Moskowitz MA (1999) Pathophysiology of ischemic stroke: an integrated view. Trends Neurosci 22:391–397
63. Xie Z, Culley DJ, Dong Y et al (2008) The common inhalation anesthetic isoflurane induces caspase activity and increases Abeta level in vivo. Ann Neurol 64:618–627
64. Lu Y, Wu X, Dong Y et al (2010) Anesthetic sevoflurane causes neurotoxicity differently in neonatal naïve and Alzheimer disease transgenic mice. Anesthesiology 112:1404–1416

Chapter 10
Mechanism of POD and POCD - Effect of Other Than Anesthetics

Shusuke Sekine and Hiroyuki Uchino

Abstract Postoperative cognitive dysfunction and delirium (POCD and POD) in adult patients of all ages and particularly the elderly are at significant risk for long-term cognitive problems. The mechanisms responsible for POCD/POD are multifactorial and the precise pathogenesis is not well known yet. Tissue injury and systemic insult associated with surgery initiate a systemic reaction accompanied by increased proinflammatory cytokines. These proinflammatory cytokines (e.g., IL-1β, IL-6, TNF-α) can induce peripheral and central nervous system (CNS) sensitization and affect hippocampal function, causing abnormal behavior, particularly memory and cognitive impairment. The inflammatory response has recently been considered a key contributor to POCD/POD.

Microglia play a key role in proinflammatory cytokine production in the CNS. The activation of microglia is tightly regulated by anti-inflammatory cytokines (e.g., IL-10, TGFβ, IL-4) to prevent a vicious cycle including microglial activation and production of proinflammatory cytokines and reactive oxygen species (ROS). Aging, chronic systemic inflammation, repetitive stress, and neurodegenerative diseases are linked to microglial priming and make microglia more sensitive to secondary challenge or insult and resistant to negative feedback. Once escaped from restrictive control, primed microglia cause an exaggerated inflammatory response and deleterious effect on the CNS leading to the development of cognitive deficits, impaired synaptic plasticity, and accelerated neurodegeneration.

Keywords POD • POCD • Immune challenge • Microglia • Oxidative stress

---

S. Sekine (✉) • H. Uchino
Department of Anesthesiology, Tokyo Medical University,
6-7-1 Nishishinjuku, Shinjuku-ku, Tokyo 160-0023, Japan
e-mail: shus@tokyo-med.ac.jp

Y. Morimoto (ed.), *Anesthesia and Neurotoxicity*,
DOI 10.1007/978-4-431-55624-4_10

10.1 Introduction

Following surgery, patients may experience cognitive decline or delirium in some cases. Postoperative delirium (POD) and cognitive dysfunction (POCD) lead to decrease in activities of daily living (ADL). They are associated with high morbidity and mortality, increased length of hospital stay, and high rates of institutionalization after discharge. It is confirmed that there is an association between delirium and long-term cognitive impairment and dementia, even after initial recovery from POD and POCD. Also, the mechanisms underlying acutely changed mental states after operations are not clear. Novel therapies are being sought that prevent or treat delirium and cognitive impairment.

Findings from animal and human studies suggest a neuroinflammatory pathogenesis of delirium and long-term brain impairment associated with critical illness and operative insult.

Here in this chapter we review research findings in animals and human beings and, from these data, formulate a hypothesis that could help to avert long-term sequelae of POD and POCD.

10.2 Risk Factors for POCD

The International Study of Post-Operative Cognitive Dysfunction (ISPOCD) found advancing age, duration of general anesthesia, lower educational level, and perioperative complications (a second operation, postoperative infections, and respiratory complications) were risk factors for early (1 week after surgery) POCD, but only age was a risk factor for late (three months after surgery) POCD. On the other hand, depth of anesthesia, hypoxia, and hypotension were not significant risk factors at any time [1].

Monk et al. found that prolonged POCD identified four independent risk factors, namely, advanced age, lower educational level, previous stroke with no residual impairment, and POCD at hospital discharge by using multiple logistic regression analysis [2]. Mild cognitive impairment (MCI) before an operation and a history of alcohol dependence are also suggested as risk factors for POCD in some studies.

In another retrospective cohort analysis, it has been demonstrated that surgery may negatively affect the domain of attention/concentration in patients with a preoperative diagnosis of MCI [3]. They suggested a correlation between POCD and MCI. In an Alzheimer's disease (AD) study, it has been demonstrated that MCI commonly preceded the onset of AD as an interim phase when there is no significant increase in senile plaques. MCI patients exhibit microglial activation and significant oxidative imbalance in comparison to age-matched controls, since the elevation of overall protein peroxidation and the oxidative modification of specific proteins are detected in the brain, including the hippocampus, and a reduction of the activity of antioxidant enzymes such as superoxide dismutase, glutathione peroxidase, and glutathione is observed in MCI patients. These facts strongly suggest that the oxidative imbalance appears at the very early stage of AD as MCI and oxidative imbalance also have a strong relationship with POCD [4].

Hudetz et al. reported that a history of alcohol dependence requiring hospitalization for detoxification in patients 55 or more years of age increased the incidence and severity of POCD after cardiac surgery using cardiopulmonary bypass (CPB) [5].

Other neuropsychological and imaging studies demonstrated dysfunction in mediofrontal and left dorsolateral prefrontal cortex in patients with chronic alcohol dependence in the absence of explicit neurological symptoms. Accordingly, neurocognitive functions might be impaired in patients with a history of alcohol dependence after cardiac surgery despite an apparent absence of preoperative neurological abnormalities.

Morimoto et al. stated that older age and low preoperative regional cerebral oxygen saturation (rSO_2) were important risk factors for postoperative delirium in patients older than 65 years of age scheduled for elective abdominal surgery [6].

Ming-hua Chen et al. measured hippocampal volume of elderly patients, who were scheduled for gastrointestinal surgery, before the operation by means of magnetic resonance imaging (MRI) scans. They showed that the hippocampal volume of the POCD group was significantly smaller than that of the non-POCD group. Therefore, hippocampal involution may have a relationship with POCD [7].

The etiology of delirium is usually considered to be multifactorial (Table 10.1). Many attempts have failed to create "universal" POD risk scales because risk factors vary widely depending on the type of intervention and the particular patient. Furthermore, such scales have been developed in the context of cardiovascular and orthopedic surgery, leaving general and emergency surgery largely underrepresented. Ansaloni et al. evaluated the incidence of POD in elderly patients undergoing general surgery and analyzed the risk factors associated with POD [8]. Delirium can be seen as the result of a complex interrelationship between predisposing factors (cognitive decline, compromised functional status, sensory impairment, pre-existing medical conditions, psychoactive drugs) and precipitating factors associated with the condition (certain drugs, primary neurological disease, intercurrent illnesses, surgery, admission to the ICU, physical restraint, and urinary catheterization) [9].

Table 10.1 Risk factors associated with postoperative delirium in elderly patients undergoing general surgery

Risk factors
Age >75 years
Comorbidity
Preoperative mild cognitive impairment
Preoperative poor functional status
Preoperative poor nutritional status
Psychopathological symptoms
Abnormal glycemic control
Secondary surgical intervention
Suboptimal postoperative care

10.3 Mechanism Responsible for POCD

As mentioned above, numerous factors contribute to the occurrence of POCD and the etiology of POCD is very complicated. It is impossible to explain the mechanism of POCD based on the type, dosage, and metabolism of specific anesthetic agents only. Numerous studies reported not only cardiac surgical procedures but also a variety of surgical procedures that have a relationship with POCD.

Postoperative neurologic deterioration is common in cardiac surgical patients, especially when cardiopulmonary bypass is used. Reduced perfusion pressure during CPB will be due to the lack of oxygen supply, which places patients at risk of cerebral ischemia. Embolization of air or particulate matter during aortic cannulation or weaning from CPB, particularly in rapid rewarming, may produce focal neurological damage and neuropsychiatric complications. CPB also causes a systemic inflammatory response, which may contribute to the development of neurologic injury. This systemic inflammation may be mediated by surgical trauma, blood contact with the extracorporeal bypass circuit, and lung reperfusion injury after discontinuation of CPB. The pathogenic mechanisms responsible for POCD remain unclear [5]. However, several studies have shown that hippocampal memory function was significantly more impaired by surgery in aged animals compared to younger control animals. This pattern has been found following a variety of surgical procedures including exploratory abdominal surgery, stabilized tibial fracture surgery, and partial hepatectomy. It is important that hippocampal memory function was demonstrated to be specifically affected by the surgical procedure and accompanying neuroinflammatory responses and not simply to the anesthetic agents administered during the surgery [10]. Numerous studies have failed to show that the mechanism of POCD depends on the type, dosage, and metabolism of specific anesthetic agents.

The central nervous system (CNS) has previously been regarded as an immune-privileged site with the absence of immune cell responses, but this dogma is not entirely true. There is a hypothesis that operative and anesthetic stress induces inflammation and it is understood that many kinds of proinflammatory cytokines (e.g., interleukin-1 beta [IL-1β], IL-6, IL-8, tumor necrotizing factor alpha [TMF-α]) are released from the surgical site occur as a first step. Cytokines released from the surgical site invade into the brain through the cerebrospinal fluid (CSF) and activate microglia in the brain. Actually, a clinical study reported that cytokine levels in CSF increased after an operation.

Microglial cells are the main cellular actors of the brain defense network and considered as the primary responders to harmful stimuli in the whole brain parenchyma. Their responses to adverse stimuli (including inflammation and stress) are mainly organized to eliminate pathogens (viruses, bacteria), phagocytizing them and cellular debris. Their functions are tissue repair and wound healing to preserve brain health [11].

A recent study revealed that microglia are also involved in the shaping of neuronal networks, contributing to neuronal activity and synaptic plasticity by a direct interaction with neurons or through the secretion of active peptides such as cytokines. Synapse formation/elimination is also a dynamic phenomenon linked to the learning and memory process. It is of concern that microglia have an active role in synapse maintenance or elimination along with directing neurogenesis in the hippocampus during adulthood.

The activation of microglia by insults or stress results in profound morphological and secreted molecular profile changes that could affect neuronal plasticity and could ultimately alter behavior. This phenomenon occurs even after an operation.

Chronic systemic inflammation also is linked to neuroinflammation by the release of proinflammatory mediators, including IL-1β, to activate microglia continuously. The primed microglia can produce an exaggerated inflammatory response in the brain, because age-dependent dysfunctions of lysosomal and mitochondrial systems allow for the hypergeneration of reactive oxygen species (ROS). The increased intracellular ROS then activates the redox-sensitive transcription factors, including nuclear factor-κ-light chain enhancer of activated B cell (NF-κB), to provoke exaggerated inflammatory responses. An inflammatory phenotype of microglia corresponded with the development of anxiety-like behavior in the repeated social defeat (RSD) model. Furthermore, changes in microglia were associated with behavioral deficits as minocycline, imipramine, and IL-1R1 antagonism prevented microglia alterations and attenuated depressive-like behavior. Specifically, it was reported that IL-1β was implicated as IL-1R1^{KO} mice and mice treated with IL-1R1 antagonist (IL-1RA) were resistant to stress-induced depressive-like behavior [11]. These results support the hypothesis that ROS and inflammatory phenomena contribute to the pathogenic mechanism of POCD [12, 13].

POCD affects a wide variety of cognitive domains, such as memory, information processing, and executive function. Learning and memory processes largely rely on the hippocampus and this brain region expresses the highest density of IL-1 receptors, making it vulnerable to the adverse consequences of neuroinflammation. A synergistic interaction between IL-1β and other cytokines, such as TNFα and IL-6, enhances this cognitive dysfunction. High levels of CNS IL-6 also inhibit memory formation and learning, cause neurodegeneration, and exacerbate sickness behavior.

Similarly, administration of lipopolysaccharide (LPS) or surgical trauma induces not only an increase in systemic cytokine level but also cytokine mRNA expression and microglial activation in the hippocampus, leading to hippocampal-dependent memory impairment. Subsequently hippocampal-dependent memory impairment after an operation was also evident in the mouse model [14–17]. In addition, subclinical infection prior to surgery may sensitize the immune system and augment the severity of POCD [16]. For example, pulmonary infection before surgery affects surgery-induced neuroinflammation and POCD in the aged rat model. Rats that had experienced mycoplasma infection before abdominal surgery and jugular vein catheterization under general anesthesia (surgery) exhibited a more generalized and exacerbated postoperative cognitive impairment compared with healthy surgery rats, as well as a prolonged increase in systemic cytokine levels and increased microglial activation in the hippocampus. These findings support the hypothesis that an infection before surgery under general anesthesia exacerbates POCD [18].

Furthermore, ketoprofen, a type of nonsteroidal anti-inflammatory drug (NSAID), or morphine inhibited an increased laparotomy-induced pain score in the postoperative pain scale. Ketoprofen could also reverse laparotomy-induced deterioration of spatial memory performance without any effect on locomotor activity and motivation. These findings indicate that effective postoperative pain management and anti-inflammatory effects with ketoprofen may have benefits for preventing the development of POCD in elderly patients [19].

10.3.1 Aging Impact on Blood-Brain Barrier

Disruption of the blood-brain barrier (BBB) is increasingly documented not only in brain vascular disease but also in aging, inflammatory conditions, and neurodegenerative disorders. To date, such evidence points mainly at an association between various dementia forms and disruption of the BBB.

Dysfunction of the BBB in the aging brain is at least in part responsible for pathological alterations such as white matter lesions, which in turn correlate with progressive cognitive deterioration. In a recent review, Farrall and Wardlaw extensively documented the increase in BBB permeability with aging in healthy individuals [20]. Different studies demonstrated significantly higher albumin leakage through the BBB in old healthy as compared to young healthy individuals, and these results were also confirmed by studies using brain imaging (computed tomography—CT, magnetic resonance imaging—MRI, or positron emission tomography—PET).

In a rodent model of senescence, morphological changes in the BBB and leakage of endogenous albumin and IgG to the brain parenchyma were selectively demonstrated for brain regions involved in cognition, such as the hippocampus. The senescence-accelerated prone mouse strain 8 (SAMP8), which shows age-related learning and memory deficits, exhibits increased oxidative stress at an early age, before other pathological features are reported. Decreased levels of superoxide dismutase and glutathione peroxidase seem to be responsible for this modification. An age-related increase in amyloid precursor protein (APP) expression without plaque formation was described in the brain of the SAMP8 mice. These results suggest that oxidative stress in brain parenchyma can trigger alterations of the BBB, possibly by cell death, gliosis, and signaling changes. Moreover, in aged Wistar rats, which show impairment in short-term memory, leakage through the BBB was found to be associated with microglial activation. The latter is a source of oxidative damage possibly not only to neurons, but also to glial and endothelial cells. Leakage of BBB can induce microglial activation by letting abnormal molecules pass into the brain parenchyma and in turn free radicals released from the microglia may further alter the BBB, in a vicious cycle. In addition, passage of neuroimmune factors to the brain also changes with senescence.

Furthermore, increased transport of TNF-α has been shown in some brain regions of old SAMP8 mice, suggesting that beyond modulating BBB properties, TNF-α is able to cross the BBB more efficiently with age. On the contrary, neurotrophin-like peptides are able to reverse this modification, suggesting that protein expression at the BBB level could be affected and protected by neurotrophins during aging.

Another effect of brain aging is the accumulation of iron in astrocytes. Iron in excess can generate free radicals and harm cells; therefore its increase in the perivascular astrocytes could play a role in alterations seen in BBB with aging, which contribute to the increase in BBB permeability [20].

10.3.2 The Aging Process Appears to Serve as a "Priming" Stimulus for Microglia, and upon Secondary Stimulation with a Triggering Stimulus

The hippocampus, which has a particularly dense microglial population, is critical for contextual and spatial learning and awareness, navigation, and episodic memories. It has been indicated that the hippocampus has been shown to exhibit higher and faster expression of proinflammatory cytokines following a peripheral immune challenge compared to other brain regions [10].

The normal aging potentiates neuroinflammatory responses to immune challenges. The majority of studies have shown that an immune challenge in aged animals induced exaggerated brain cytokine responses causing impairments in long-term memory [10].

Observations made in animals and in human brain tissue indicate that microglia become overactivated with advancing age and that aging causes amplified cytokine production after subsequent challenges, even if these challenges are not strong. In addition, various surgical procedures have been reported to produce an IL-1β increase in the hippocampus of aged animals for up to several days compared to age-matched sham controls. In contrast, young adult animals that underwent the same surgical procedure showed no differences in IL-1β expression compared to their age-matched sham controls. Effects of peripheral inflammation on the brain are most distinct in animals with chronic neurodegeneration and increase with the aging process. These results indicate chronic neurodegeneration with the aging process makes microglia more sensitive and overactivated to subsequent immune challenge.

Similarly to age effects on microglial cytokine expression profile, there is increased expression of inflammatory markers including MHC II and complement receptor 3 (CD11b) in the aged brain of humans, rodents, canines, and nonhuman primates. Many of these markers are present specifically on microglia in the aged brain, including MHC II [17].

Immune challenge in the aged leads to exaggerated proinflammatory cytokine production by microglia. For example, pretreatment with minocycline, an anti-inflammatory agent and reported microglial inhibitor, attenuated the LPS-induced amplification of TLR2, IL-1β, IL-6, and the inflammatory associated enzyme indoleamine 2,3-dioxygenase (IDO), which reduce serotonin production in the hippocampus of aged mice.

Proinflammatory cytokines activate IDO. As a result, the amount of serotonin production will decrease. Proinflammatory cytokines also activate the serotonin transporter leading to lack of serotonin. A paucity of serotonin exacerbates depression.

Moreover, a recent study showed that MHC II positive microglia were responsible for the robust increase in IL-1β following inter-peritoneal (i.p.) injection of LPS. In this study, LPS-treated aged mice had a significant increase in MHC II positive microglia expressing IL-1β. Furthermore, additional analysis of microglia from aged mice indicated that 95% of MHC II positive microglia were IL-1β positive. MHC II is considered a marker for primed microglia. For this reason, these data support the hypothesis that primed MHC II positive microglia are highly responsive to immune challenge and provide a direct connection between heightened neuroinflammation and microglia, particularly in the aged population.

CD68 is widely recognized as a marker for microglial activation, similarly to MHC II. In a post-mortem case-control study, CD68 expression on microglia was increased in elderly patients with sepsis. This increase was accompanied by raised numbers of amoeboid-formed microglia in grey matter, indicating an enhanced immunological response in human brain tissue during a systemic inflammatory reaction. De-ramified morphological alteration is comparable to the activation of microglia.

The microglial response is usually tightly regulated to prevent deleterious effects; however, this inflammatory response has the potential to become self-amplifying. Once microglia escape from strict control, their defensive features might turn neurotoxic. A self-propelling neuroinflammatory reaction in the brain is initiated by systemic inflammation that can persist for months. Circulating cytokines released as the result of an inflammatory response can cross the BBB and activate resting microglia or cause an exaggerated inflammatory response in primed microglia [21]. Ultimately, this inflammatory response can become associated with cognitive impairments or even dementia. These results indicate that the neuroinflammation is both exaggerated and prolonged especially in the aged brain compared to the young animal model following central or peripheral stimulation.

Repeated stress exposure causes deregulation of neuroendocrine and neuroimmune pathways that increase neuroinflammatory responses negatively affecting cognition and behavior. Several models of aging indicate that aging causes changes in microglial response. An exaggerated and prolonged cytokine response is associated with the development of cognitive, behavioral, and physiological complications that are interpreted to be maladaptive to the host organism [17]. Chronic low-grade inflammation was shown to exacerbate postoperative (neuro)inflammation as well as postoperative cognitive impairment in both rodent models and clinical studies. Aging has a strong relationship with repeated stress exposure (e.g., chronic inflammatory disease, many chances to be sensitized to microorganisms, and chronic pain). Consistent with prolonged stress exposure leading to increased neuroinflammatory signaling, microglia have robust changes in morphology and are activated, which may contribute to the neurobiology underlying mood and cognitive disturbances. Neuroinflammation is responsible for mood and cognitive disorder also in the postoperative phase.

10.3.3 Acetylcholine Can Inhibit Release of the Proinflammatory Cytokines and Vagus Nerve Stimulation Inhibits Systemic Inflammation

Systemic infection and anticholinergic effects of drug treatment are both recognized risk factors for delirium. Findings of experimental studies show that chronic low-dose LPS infusion in rats produces extensive neuroinflammation and a substantial reduction in cortical choline acetyltransferase activity as a marker of cholinergic integrity. Vagus nerve stimulation inhibits systemic inflammation and acetylcholine can inhibit the release of the proinflammatory cytokines TNFα and IL- 1 and 6 in human endotoxin-stimulated macrophages. Although the mechanisms underlying these anti-inflammatory effects are not known exactly, a major role of the spleen has been suggested, because splenectomy has been shown to prevent anti-inflammatory effects of vagus nerve stimulation. These experiments have paved the way for the idea of a cholinergic anti-inflammatory pathway, by which the brain senses and modulates the systemic inflammatory response through the vagus nerve. Analogous to what has been noted in peripheral tissues, acetylcholine seems to also have a role in control of brain inflammation. Microglia express nicotinic receptors and activation of these cholinergic receptors attenuates the proinflammatory response in vitro [22]. These results suggest that vagus nerve stimulation and acetylcholine may inhibit microglial activation and prevent the onset of POCD and POD.

10.3.4 Noradrenergic Pathways Appear to Affect the Motility and Morphology of Microglia During Inflammatory Conditions

Microglia express α1, α2, β1, and β2-adrenergic receptors. Moreover, noradrenergic neurons originating in the locus coeruleus (LC) project to several brain regions that demonstrate microglial activation induced by RSD. Indeed, pretreatment with propranolol, a β-adrenergic receptor antagonist, reduced neuronal and microglial activation in stress-responsive brain regions and prevented the development of anxiety. Other reports revealed that central administration of β-adrenergic receptor agonists alone can elicit proinflammatory cytokine production. Furthermore, ablation of noradrenergic LC projections is shown to reduce stress-induced IL-1β production. These results indicate that central noradrenergic responses have a substantial contribution to neuroinflammatory signaling via stress-induced microglial activation [11].

10.3.5 The Concept of "Microglial Aging"

This concept is based on the fact that sensitized microglia are the key contributor to the acceleration of cognitive decline, which is the major sign of brain aging. On the other hand, long-lasting elevations in proinflammatory cytokines in the hippocampus produce memory impairments [10]. Inflammation induces oxidative stress and DNA damage, which leads to the overproduction of ROS by numerous types of cells, including macrophages and microglia. Oxidative stress-damaged cells successively produce larger amounts of inflammatory mediators to promote microglial aging.

Microglia, the resident mononuclear phagocytes in the brain, are chronically or pathologically activated to affect the neuronal environment. There is increasing evidence that activated microglia produce excessive ROS during aging and hypoxia, resulting in the NF-κB dependent excessive production of proinflammatory mediators, including IL-1β, TNF-α, and IL-6. Furthermore, activated microglia-mediated neuroinflammation is closely associated with the pathogenesis of Alzheimer's disease (AD), because activated microglia trigger neuroinflammation to promote neuronal damage and the deposition of amyloid β (Aβ). Cognitive decline is a main symptom of AD. There may be similarities among POD, COPD, and AD. It is already known that the CNS dysfunction attended with AD may increase the risk for the development of POCD [23]. Injection of Aβ into the lateral ventricle of the mouse brain is known to create an animal model of AD, which has been reported to result in learning and memory dysfunction, decline of choline acetyltransferase activity, and inhibition of long-term potentiation (LTP) induction. The symptoms of AD are classified into core symptoms, such as cognitive dysfunction, and behavioral psychological symptoms of dementia (BPSD), including excitation, aggressiveness, hallucination, delusion, apathy, disinterest, anxiety, and depression. Cognitive dysfunction and BPSD are thought to be associated with neurofunctional and neuropathological abnormalities in the brain. BPSD-like behavior is observed in postoperative patients, which is similar to POD symptoms. Moreover, Aβ causes not only an increase in the extracellular concentration of glutamate but also inhibition of glutamate uptake by astrocytes. Proinflammatory mediators such as IL-1β also severely impair glutamate transport, further exacerbating disease states. As a result, excess of extracellular glutamate concentration causes glutamate excitotoxicity, which is a final common pathway for neuronal death, and observed in numerous pathological processes such as stroke/ischemia and temporal lobe epilepsy. It is known that glutamate is toxic to cultured neuronal cells via two different processes, both of which result in the production of free radicals. The classical pathway, known as excitotoxicity, occurs through the activation of NMDA and non-NMDA glutamatergic receptors and subsequent calcium influx into the cells. Kawakami et al. confirmed that an increase in the extracellular level of glutamate and degeneration of neuronal and astroglial cells were observed in the brain of thiamine-deficient (TD) rats, and found that TJ-54, a traditional herbal medicine, inhibited not only the TD-induced increase in extracellular level of glutamate but also the degeneration of cerebral neurocytes and astrocytes in the vulnerable brain regions. BPSD-like behaviors such as anxiety, depression, muricide, attacking, and startle responses, as well as impairment of learning and memory, are observed in TD rats and mice. *Uncaria rhynchophylla*, a constituent herb of TJ-54, was shown to protect against NMDA-induced neuronal excitotoxicity in rat hippocampus or to block NMDA-induced current in cortical neurons. TJ-54 bound strongly to glutamate and glycine recognition sites in NMDA receptors and protected against glutamate-induced cell death [24].

As the stimulation of NMDA receptors by glutamate induces an intracellular Ca^{2+} overload and activates neuronal NOS, resulting in excessive production of NO and formation of ROS and lipid peroxidation to induce neuronal death, so, too, does IL-6 exposure substantially increasing intracellular calcium and sensitizing neurons to excitatory stimulation. On the other hand, anti-inflammatory agents improve the cognitive functions of AD patients. Besides, it is also well accepted that chronic systemic inflammation can alter the neuroinflammation in the brain. A clinical study has demonstrated the impact of rheumatoid arthritis (RA) and periodontitis on AD, and recent experimental studies have clarified the routes of inflammatory signal transduction from chronic systemic inflammation to the brain and microglial priming. Aging also has been associated with a chronic low-grade increase in systemic and central inflammatory markers. Hence, these results suggest that immune challenges and chronic low-grade inflammation during life cause age-related alterations in the immune environment of the body and brain. Life events, such as chronic inflammatory disease, infection, and physical trauma, may thus contribute to an exacerbated neuroinflammatory response to surgery and might therefore be associated with the susceptibility to POCD. Accordingly, preoperative depression, metabolic syndrome, and a secondary surgical intervention increase the risk of POCD [8].

10.3.6 Impaired Regulation of Microglia in the Aged Brain

The cause of this amplified microglial activation with age may be related to impairments in several key regulatory systems that make it more difficult to resolve microglial activation. The activation of microglia is tightly regulated by anti-inflammatory cytokines including IL-10, TGFβ, and IL-4, which decrease in the brain with age (Fig. 10.1). Activated microglia from aged brain are refractory to anti-inflammatory stimulus.

IL-10 is a potent anti-inflammatory cytokine that should regulate IL-1β production and decrease inflammation. However, IL-10 was decreased in the brain of aged rodents under homeostatic conditions.

TGFβ increases fractalkine receptor expression and reduces IL-1β mRNA in BV2 microglial cell lines stimulated with LPS. BV2 microglial cell lines have been established primarily by in vitro models used to study neuroinflammation for more than a decade. Fractalkine is important in maintaining functional plasticity of

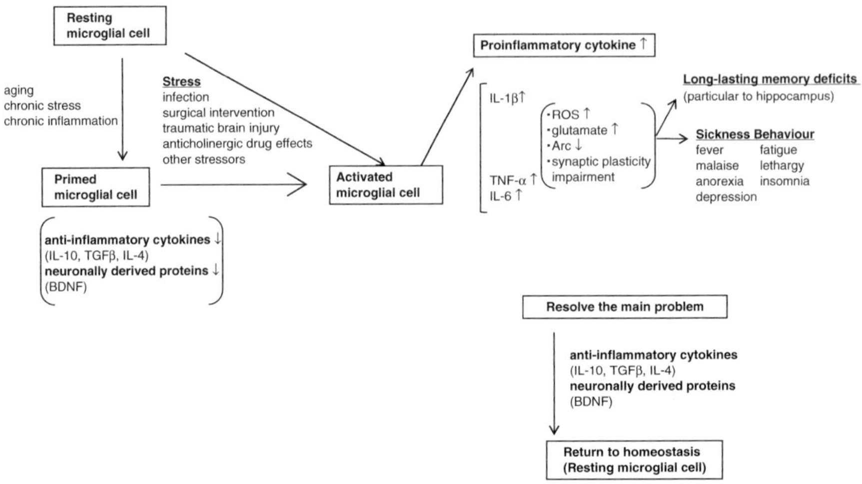

Fig. 10.1 Microglia hypothesis of POCD. Primed microglia cause exaggerated and prolonged neuroinflammatory responses, which correlate with long-lasting memory deficit. This amplified response is particular to the hippocampus. Stress events and life events stimulate resting microglia and can increase the primed microglial population. Primed microglia prepare for subsequent inflammatory challenge. Microglial activity can be modulated and shut off by anti-inflammatory cytokines and neuronally derived proteins, which are reduced in the aged brain

microglia. Decreases in either the ligand or receptor can lead microglia to be activated. In adult mice, TGFβ mRNA increased in the brain 24 h after LPS injection; however, this increase was not detected in aged mice. This lack of TGFβ mRNA induction following inflammatory challenge can therefore be a possible link to the prolonged microglial activation reported in aged mice.

IL-4 is another anti-inflammatory cytokine that is affected by age. It has been indicated that there are reductions in IL-4 with age; there are also reductions in IL-4 sensitivity with age in the animal model. Following IL-4 challenge, microglia from adult mice shifted in phenotype toward an alternatively activated M2 state, in which microglia play roles in anti-neuroinflammation. On the other hand, microglia from aged mice retained a classically activated M1 phenotype that contributes to inflammation, even in the presence of IL-4. Induction of hippocampal IL-4 successfully restored LTP in the aged rats suggesting an important role for IL-4 to modulate the CNS environment and retain LTP by lowering CNS inflammation. Either reduced levels of IL-4 or a reduced sensitivity to IL-4 in the aged brain impairs the ability to lower inflammation in the brain. This is potentially important because IL-4 has a role in maintaining memory and learning, reparative processes after traumatic CNS injury, and also affects the regulation of microglial activity.

Taken together, deficits in IL-10, TGFβ, and IL-4 signaling pathways with age may lead to a reduced ability to regulate and shut off microglia, which contributes to lower inflammation, modulates the CNS environment, and maintains the learning and memory function [17].

10.4 Mitochondrial Dysfunction Effect on Neuronal Impairment

Mitochondrial dysfunction leads to impaired bioenergetics, decrease in adenosine-5′-triphosphate (ATP) production, impaired calcium homeostasis, increased production of free radicals, and oxidative stress. It is also involved in neuronal development, synaptogenesis, synaptic development, and plasticity. In microglia, mitochondrial dysfunction leads to the excess production of ROS, which promotes the redox imbalance and stimulates proinflammatory gene transcription and the release of cytokines, such as IL-1, IL-6, and TNF-α, thereby inducing neuroinflammation. ROS are part of the neuroinflammatory cascade and can play a prominent role in the development of age-related declines in LTP, cognition, sickness behaviors, and other neuronal functions. On the other hand, several studies suggest that dietary supplements high in antioxidants may be an effective treatment in buffering against age-related neuroinflammatory-induced cognitive impairment. It is important to maintain antioxidant levels and control ROS activity. For example, neuroinflammatory prolonged oxidative stress leads to the accumulation of Aβ and tau phosphorylation and then induces neurotoxicity and cognitive impairment in AD patients. The inflammatory cell-mediated overproduction of TNF-α is thought to be the main contributor to the increased release of ROS in RA patients, because TNF-α not only causes cell damage but also inhibits antioxidants, such as superoxide dismutase 1 (SOD1) and SOD3 [4]. Numerous studies have indicated excess ROS levels and the depletion of antioxidant levels in the gingival crevicular fluid. There is further evidence of higher levels of lipid peroxidation, hydrogen peroxides, and oxidative DNA damage in animal models. Therefore, ROS promote oxidative damage, modulate the intracellular and extracellular redox status, and interfere with the activation of proteolytic enzymes in the systemic inflammatory environment, leading to neurotoxicity and cognitive impairment.

Stress, including systemic insult or genetic defects, can cause mitochondrial dysfunction, which leads to increased oxidative stress and/or altered calcium homeostasis. An excess of glutamate in the synapse leads to an excess of cytosolic calcium, which produces overactivity of calcium-dependent enzymes and an overload of mitochondria by calcium; it leads to cytoskeletal degradation, protein malformation, decrease in ATP production, and increase in oxygen radical generation. Different stimuli, such as hypoxia/ischemia, seizure, and hypoglycemia, all activate this pathway. These processes can lead to atrophy or death of neurons, which are related to neuroinflammatory-induced cognitive impairment.

10.5 POCD Prevention

As mentioned above, neuroinflammation is involved in POCD and it is supposed that modulating inflammation contributes to prevention and treatment of POCD.

Administration of IL-1 receptor antagonist (IL-1RA) prior to a peripheral *E. coli* infection or abdominal surgery prevented the *E. coli* and surgery-induced suppression of activity-dependent cytoskeletal-associated protein (Arc), increases in IL-6, hippocampal IL-1β increases, and long-lasting long-term memory (LTM) impairments. These results suggest that preventing the cascade of neuroinflammatory sequelae especially in the aged brain may protect against the deleterious effects of the otherwise unrestrained inflammatory response following a challenge.

Chapman et al. also examined the effects of IL-1RA. They found that a single central administration of IL-1RA, at the time of a peripheral *E. coli* injection, abrogated the aging-associated, infection-induced impairment of theta-burst late phase-LTP in hippocampal area 1. Theta waves are observed in the hippocampus of unanesthetized awake animals [10]. Consistent with these findings, Abraham and Johnson reported that central administration of IL-1RA blocks LPS-induced sickness behaviors in aged mice [10]. These studies provide evidence that alterations to hippocampal microglial phenotype and an exaggerated proinflammatory cytokine response play an important role in their cognitive health following an immune challenge in aged animals.

Therefore, pharmacological interventions that control microglial activation states hold considerable promise with regard to neuroinflammatory-induced memory impairments in the aged and postoperative population.

Minocycline, a second-generation semi-synthetic tetracycline derivative, has been recognized as an anti-inflammatory, neuroprotective, and anti-apoptotic agent in several animal models such as stroke, traumatic brain injury, and spinal cord injury, as well as several animal models of neurodegenerative disease. Moreover, it has also been reported that minocycline reduced microglial activation and spatial learning and memory impairment after hypoglycemic brain injury as well as attenuated the age-related increase in hippocampal IL-1β, while partially restoring deficits in LTP. Pretreating aged animals with minocycline reduced the hippocampal proinflammatory response to LPS. Furthermore, minocycline was also demonstrated to be effective at improving surgery-induced and isoflurane-induced memory impairments in aged rodents. Therefore, these effects are thought to arise through the inhibition of microglial activation and modulation of cytokine expression [25].

Amantadine has been found to have significant neuroprotective effects. One of the mechanisms for these effects is to enhance the production of glial cell line-derived neurotrophic factor (GDNF) as shown in cell culture studies. GDNF, a cloned member of the transforming growth factor-beta (TGFβ) superfamily, can inhibit microglial activation and neuroinflammation. Deficits in TGFβ and IL-10 signaling pathways with age may lead to a reduced ability to shut off microglia [17]. Amantadine attenuated surgery-induced learning and memory impairment. GDNF blocks surgery-induced cognitive impairment. In several studies it has been shown to induce IL-1β levels in the hippocampus and has also been shown to robustly decrease brain-delivered neurotrophic factor (BDNF), a member of the neurotrophin family of growth factors, mRNA in the hippocampus, and resulted in hippocampal-dependent memory deficits. On the contrary, intrahippocampal administration of IL-1RA prevented both the BDNF mRNA downregulation and the memory impairments produced by the immune challenge [10].

Amantadine inhibited the expression of ionized calcium binding adapter molecule 1 (Iba-1), a microglial marker, IL-1β, and IL-6 in the hippocampus, and the translocation of p65, a NF-κB component, into nuclei of the microglia in the hippocampus; all of them were induced by surgery. On the contrary, anti-GDNF antibody inhibited amantadine-induced attenuation of learning and memory impairment after surgery. Surgery induces neuroinflammation and amantadine increases GDNF in the brain and reduces these surgical effects. GDNF reduces inflammatory cytokine production from microglia and antagonizing GDNF reverses the effects of amantadine on surgery-induced cognitive dysfunction. Consequently, it is supposed that amantadine attenuates the surgery-induced neuroinflammation and cognitive impairment by means of increasing GDNF and modulating neuroinflammation in the animal model, which contributes to preventing POD and POCD [26].

Recently, many studies in aged animals have reported robust effects of physical exercise on hippocampal neurogenesis and hippocampal memory performance. Running restored presynaptic density and neurogenesis in the hippocampus optimized intrahippocampal neuronal connectivity and reversed the aging-associated memory deficits in the hippocampal-dependent task of place recognition. Physical exercise has been extensively shown to strongly increase BDNF mRNA and protein levels in the hippocampus and decreased IL-1β production. Given the prominent role of BDNF in learning and memory processes, the effects of exercise-induced BDNF in aged animals are of great interest. Moreover, small amounts of voluntary exercise in aged rats were an effective therapeutic intervention to prevent *E. coli*-induced BDNF blunting, neuroinflammatory responses, and long-term memory impairments. With important implications for reducing the neuroinflammatory response, exercise has also been demonstrated to modulate the activation state of microglia and to prevent hippocampal microglial priming, with recent evidence suggesting that this protection may occur through the exercise-induced downregulation of glucocorticoid receptors (GRs) in the hippocampus. Furthermore, in an AD mouse model, increased levels of BDNF and markers for neuroprotection and plasticity were exhibited after 6 months of voluntary wheel running. This amount of exercise was also associated with activated antioxidant signaling pathways and protected against cognitive decline and dementia-like behaviors. There is a tremendous amount of evidence to support thc beneficial effects of exercise for hippocampal function and thus cognitive health in the aged population with chronic neuroinflammation. Physical exercise is the only way to prevent delirium even in the critical care setting. This mechanism applies equally to the postoperative phase.

References

1. Moller JT, Cluitmans P, Rasmussen LS et al (1998) Long-term postoperative cognitive dysfunction in the elderly ISPOCD1 study. ISPOCD investigators. International study of postoperative cognitive dysfunction. Lancet 21:857–861
2. Monk TG, Weldon BC, Garvan CW et al (2008) Predictors of cognitive dysfunction after major noncardiac surgery. Anesthesiology 108:18–30
3. Bekker A, Lee C, de Santi S et al (2010) Does mild cognitive impairment increase the risk of developing postoperative cognitive dysfunction? Am J Surg 199:782–788
4. Wu Z, Yu J, Zhu A et al (2016) Nutrients, microglia aging, and brain aging. Oxidative Med Cell Longev 2016:7498528. doi:10.1155/2016/7498528
5. Hudetz JA, Patterson KM, Byrne AJ et al (2009) A history of alcohol dependence increases the incidence and severity of postoperative cognitive dysfunction in cardiac surgical patients. Int J Environ Res Public Health 6:2725–2739
6. Morimoto Y, Yoshimura M, Utada K et al (2009) Prediction of postoperative delirium after abdominal surgery in the elderly. J Anesth 23:51–56
7. Chen MH, Liao Y, Rong PF et al (2013) Hippocampal volume reduction in elderly patients at risk for postoperative cognitive dysfunction. J Anesth 27:487–492
8. Ansaloni L, Catena F, Chattat R et al (2010) Risk factors and incidence of postoperative delirium in elderly patients after elective and emergency surgery. Br J Surg 97:273–280
9. Ganai S, Lee KF, Merrill A et al (2007) Adverse outcomes of geriatric patients undergoing abdominal surgery who are at high risk for delirium. Arch Surg 142:1072–1078
10. Barrientos RM, Kitt MM, Watkins LR et al (2015) Neuroinflammation in the normal aging hippocampus. Neuroscience 309:84–99
11. Delpech JC, Madore C, Nadjar A et al (2015) Microglia in neuronal plasticity: influence of stress. Neuropharmacology 96:19–28
12. Buvanendran A, Kroin JS, Berger RA et al (2006) Upregulation of prostaglandin E2 and interleukins in the central nervous system and peripheral tissue during and after surgery in humans. Anesthesiology 104:403–410
13. Peng L, Xu L, Ouyang W (2013) Role of peripheral inflammatory markers in postoperative cognitive dysfunction (POCD): a meta-analysis. PLoS One 8:e79624
14. Terrando N, Rei FA, Vizcaychipi M et al (2010) The impact of IL-1 modulation on the development of lipopolysaccharide-induced cognitive dysfunction. Crit Care 14:R88
15. Cibelli M, Fidalgo AR, Terrando N et al (2010) Role of interleukin-1beta in postoperative cognitive dysfunction. Ann Neurol 68:360–368
16. Fidalgo AR, Cibelli M, White JP et al (2011) Systemic inflammation enhances surgery-induced cognitive dysfunction in mice. Neurosci Lett 498:63–66
17. Norden DM, Godbout JP (2013) Microglia of the aged brain: primed to be activated and resistant to regulation. Neuropathol Appl Neurobiol 39:19–34
18. Hovens IB, van Leeuwen BL, Nyakas C et al (2015) Prior infection exacerbates postoperative cognitive dysfunction in aged rats. Am J Physiol Regul Integr Comp Physiol 309:R148–R159
19. Kawano T, Takahashi T, Iwata H et al (2014) Effects of ketoprofen for prevention of postoperative cognitive dysfunction in aged rats. J Anesth 28:932–936
20. Popescu BO, Toescu EC, Popescu LM et al (2009) Blood-brain barrier alterations in ageing and dementia. J Neurol Sci 283:99–106
21. Morandi A, Hughes CG, Girard TD et al (2011) Statins and brain dysfunction: a hypothesis to reduce the burden of cognitive impairment in patients who are critically ill. Chest 140:580–585
22. van Gool WA, van de Beek D, Eikelenboom P (2010) Systemic infection and delirium: when cytokines and acetylcholine collide. Lancet 375:773–775
23. Evered L, Silbert B, Scott DA et al (2016) Cerebrospinal fluid biomarker for Alzheimer disease predicts postoperative cognitive dysfunction. Anesthesiology 124:353–361

24. Kawakami Z, Kanno H, Ueki T et al (2009) Neuroprotective effects of yokukansan, a traditional Japanese medicine, on glutamate-mediated excitotoxicity in cultured cells. Neuroscience 159:1397–1407
25. Won SJ, Kim JH, Yoo BH et al (2012) Prevention of hypoglycemia-induced neuronal death by minocycline. J Neuroinflammation 9:225. doi:10.1186/1742-2094-9-225
26. Zhang J, Tan H, Jiang W et al (2014) Amantadine alleviates postoperative cognitive dysfunction possibly by increasing glial cell line-derived neurotrophic factor in rats. Anesthesiology 121:773–785

MIX
Papier aus verantwortungsvollen Quellen
Paper from responsible sources
FSC® C105338

If you have any concerns about our products,
you can contact us on
ProductSafety@springernature.com

In case Publisher is established outside the EU,
the EU authorized representative is:
Springer Nature Customer Service Center GmbH
Europaplatz 3, 69115 Heidelberg, Germany

Printed by Libri Plureos GmbH
in Hamburg, Germany